Minding yourSELF

Dave Nixon

....

MINDING
yourSELF

....

Clear the crap.

**Take back your life
through Mindset,
Movement, & Nutrition.**

MEYER & MEYER SPORT

British Library Cataloguing in Publication Data
A catalogue record for this book is available from the British Library

Minding yourSELF
Maidenhead: Meyer & Meyer Sport (UK) Ltd., 2020
ISBN: 978-1-78255-188-1

Aachen, Auckland, Beirut, Cairo, Cape Town, Dubai, Hägendorf, Hong Kong, India-napolis, Manila, New Delhi, Singapore, Sydney, Tehran, Vienna

 Member of the World Sports Publishers' Association (WSPA), www.w-s-p-a.org
Printed by C-M Books, Ann Arbor, MI
ISBN: 978-1-78255-188-1
Email: info@m-m-sports.com
www.thesportspublisher.com

CONTENTS

FOREWORD

I have had the distinct pleasure to know Dave Nixon for several years. He originally started off as a client of mine and immediately struck me as a really smart and knowledgeable individual. I've also had the chance to meet and hang out with Dave in person, which is saying something because he lives in Australia, and I live in the US. Dave made a trip to the US a couple of years ago, and we've still connected frequently through email, podcasts, in person, and numerous video calls. I am honored to be a part of his book and, in particular, his larger vision for health that covers not only the physical component, but the mental aspect as well.

Too many times books offer all sorts of great advice, but at the same time, they miss some key practical elements. This book is different, and Dave really does a great job of exploring how the mental and physical aspects of health and fitness go together. It's sometimes far too easy to get caught up in being so precise with diet and training that the practical component is overlooked. During my many conversations with Dave over the years, he's always telling me that "XYZ" might be great in theory, but it's utterly meaningless unless you can take that information and package it into an easy-to-digest format. That's what Dave sets out to do in this book.

It was my pleasure to help write the nutrition component of this book. My main goal was to cover some of the intricacies of nutrition, but at the same time make sure things are packaged in that easy-to-digest manner that Dave is all about. Through my company, Renaissance Periodization, we have helped hundreds of thousands of clients across the world in the last six years. We can talk all of the nitty gritty details of the science behind diet and training. Where we align great with Dave is that most of that is not going to actually help clients. What actually does help clients is breaking it down into the simplest and easy to understand way possible, which we do through simplifying things through our RP Diet App and diet templates.

If you're looking for a book that will cut through all the nonsense out there in the fitness world and will leave you with some solid, practical tips to become an all-around healthier YOU, then read this book. It's not just about fitness, it's about balancing everything—training, nutrition, recovery, and mental health. It may be great to be a rock star in any one of those areas or, heck, even two or three. Missing any of the elements will leave a big gap in your personal self, and Dave's aim is to help you fill this gap. He wants you to become better at everything, and his book will help you get there. By becoming better in every single one of those areas, you'll discover more about yourself than you ever thought possible. By becoming more self-aware and truly understanding all parts of yourself, then you will truly be on the right journey in life.

I hope you get as much out of this book as I did, and we welcome your feedback. Thank you!

–Nick Shaw
CEO and co-founder of Renaissance Periodization

PREFACE

I wrote this book knowing that it isn't for everyone. In fact, you could argue that is why I wrote it because those who I've written the book for will feel like I wrote it especially for them.

The super interesting thing about this book is that someone may read it at one point in their life, and it may not make any sense at all, only to read it again two, three or even eight years later and have it become a catalyst for an absolutely breathtaking moment of clarity. One of my favourite quotes is, "no man steps in the same river twice, for its not the same river and he's not the same man".

The information in this book may hit you like a tonne of bricks, like it did me at some point when I learned it. Or maybe it won't, because it isn't for you. Yet. Maybe the information in this book are already tattooed on the inside of your brain. If that's the case, congratulations. You see life in a way many do not.

This book was written for the renegades. The individuals. Those who seek a life in the fields out past the towns of mediocrity. Those who know greatness lies sleeping within.

Did you know that the most beautiful thing about greatness is just how different it looks on everyone? Different or not, it is there, and this book was written to help you wake your sleeping greatness. For we are nothing but potential, and more often than not, it is not about speeding up the river of potential in order to try and get to where you want, but rather remove the rocks that block its flow. This is why I wrote this book. So we can remove our own rocks that we have in the way of our potential. So we can identify them, see them for once and for all, and then over time, one by one, remove them so our potential can flow again.

When I started writing this book, the goal was to give you, the reader, a fully integrated and holistic approach to health in a way that was both consumable and practical. Interestingly enough, what I actually wrote was slightly different. Although I covered the three main areas of health (mindset, movement, and nutrition), I ended up heavily writing this from a developmental standpoint. That simply means what I offer in this book in terms of fitness and nutrition is heavily seen through the lens of our mindset towards those two areas of health.

There is already so much objective advice and books out there on what to eat, what exercise program to do, and why it's better than all of the others. I didn't want this book to be that. I wanted this book to be a meta to that. To see it from a different lens. Though we have more doctors, more nutritionists, more gyms, the highest access to food and information ever, yet we are still unhealthy and unhappy means that something needs to change.

So this book won't give you the exact right diet or tell you how to think, and it won't give you a training plan. What this book will do is equip you with knowledge so that you know where to look.

I have outlined the three main areas of health and then provided a map for how to measure your progress through all three areas. I have taken a completely different approach compared to the traditional model of fitness and health. I have taken the focus off the program and the diet and instead put it on what you want to achieve with your life. Once you have established that, then we make sure the training (both mental and physical) and nutritional programs are set up in a way that will support that.

Simple. Not easy, but simple.

And although I don't share training programs and diet plans, there are links and references for recommended online resources for mental development, physical training and nutritional programming. Still, health isn't a one size fits all. That is why I wrote this book. So people can improve their Health IQ. Or become what I call, BossFit.

Did you know that the word "boss" is derived from the Dutch word "baas" which practically translates to "master"?

To be BossFit means to be your own master. To master your mind, master your craft, and ultimately master your life. To be free of unnecessary suffering and struggle. To live life within your power and on your terms.

I originally wrote the draft using the term Health IQ but after much deliberation, I realised that Health IQ is the map we use in order to measure where we are and where we need to get to. I decided to leave Health IQ in there and let BossFit become a project of its own. Maybe even an extension of this book at a later date. That aside, if you follow the guidelines outlined in this book, set clearly defined targets, commit to training your mind, your body, and educate yourself about food, you will become BossFit.

You will master your life. But you have to start by minding your*self*. I hope this book challenges you in ways that help you grow.

See you on the other side.

ACKNOWLEDGMENTS

Reading through book acknowledgments in the past, I thought they were only a bunch of names people felt the need to mention. It never really occurred to me what goes into putting a book together. Being on the other side now as the author, I can assure you that writing a book is a team effort. I have nothing but gratitude for the amazing people that were a part of my team with this book.

To the crew at Pubilshizer who helped get my idea off the ground and helped me put a proposal together and land a world-class publisher, thank you.

To every single person who pre-ordered a book and supported me when this was still just a thought, thank you from the bottom of my heart.

To the team at Meyer & Meyer Sport, thank you for the opportunity and patience with working with me. Especially Liz, you have been an absolute gem, and this book wouldn't have lived up to its potential without you.

To my team and family at Functional Fitness Australia, thank you for your patience, support and love. You guys are a part of my home.

To my beautiful, caring, supportive, loving fiancée, thank you with all of my being.

To Peaty, my Mini Schnauzer puppy, you were a massive distraction, and you have no idea how hard I am working so you can have a bigger backyard to bark at nothing in particular. (P.S. I love you.)

To everyone reading, this book is a piece of my soul and a time stamp of where I am and unfolding as a human at this moment, and thank you for sharing that with me.

Big Love,
Dave

INTRODUCTION
THE HUMAN MOVEMENT

Before reviewing the title of this book and settling on *Minding yourSELF,* the book was originally called *The Human Movement* (a.k.a. *THM*). *THM* came from a concept I had called "Training for the Zombie Apocalypse."

So the better question to start may be where did "Training for the Zombie Apocalypse" come from? (Let's call it T4ZA.)

No, it wasn't *The Walking Dead, Dawn of the Dead, Night of the Living Dead,* or anything dead for that matter. It came from the idea that in today's world it is the drinks we drink, the food we eat, the drugs we take, and the way we move or, more importantly, the way we don't move that is actually eating our brains. Add that to too many hours watching horror movies or the news (kind of the same thing really), some solid text neck, and arthritis in our thumbs from swiping, and we start to realize that maybe the apocalypse isn't sometime in the future or some fictional narrative; maybe, just maybe, it is happening right here, right now all around us.

You see, we are the zombies. Living right now. Well, kind of living. More like existing. Always building a future in anticipation for the future so that when we arrive in the future, we won't be living in that moment because we will be too busy preparing for the future.

Think about it. Living doesn't happen in the future; it happens right now. Here, in this very moment.

Now this is not to say that you shouldn't save for the future or sacrifice some of the present to set up a future. What I am referring to is that there is a high chance that you don't want to look back on your life and realize you spent it preparing to live rather than living it. There's a way to balance this, which I know varies for each individual, and I don't necessarily have a specific and clear answer for that in this book. What I do have for you in this book is a map that you can use to navigate you toward LIVING your best life, a map you can use to train for the zombie apocalypse.

I call this map the Health IQ Map.

Back in November of 2014, I reached out to speak to Simon Sinek, author of *Start with Why* (among other great titles). His team responded and said that he wasn't in a position to talk with every person who requested it and instead put me in touch with a guy by the name of Stephen Shedletzky. Stephen was one of Simon's right-hand men.

(For those of you who don't know Simon, go watch his TED Talk "How Great Leaders Inspire Action.")

When talking with Stephen, I shared my concept of T4ZA, and he had one bit of advice for me. That bit of advice had been passed from Simon to him when he mentioned he wanted to write a book called *Marketing Is a Dirty Word* (from memory—sorry if I have paraphrased your title, Stephen).

Simon encouraged him to state his title in the positive. Effectively, give it a name that doesn't just go with the fashions of the day but one that will be historically true and stand the test of time. It was this bit of advice that transformed T4ZA into something with much more meaning and significance.

It turned training for the zombie apocalypse into the human movement, and in order for the human movement to occur, we truly need to be minding ourselves.

Why I Broke Up With the Health and Fitness Industry

I originally had this later in the book but decided to bring this topic forward earlier on because it will help people understand why I take the angle I take and why I may sound different to others in the fitness and health industry.

My career in the fitness industry started at the age of 15. I was a quiet young boy behind the desk of a local gym in Canberra, Australia, doing some admin work. Like many young males (and I know young females go through their own version of this), I was wanting to get big. To prove something. So that people noticed me. Growing up playing team sports such as cricket and Australian Rules Football, I enjoyed being around people; that was certain. But the reality is that as a teenager I wanted to get as big as possible because that was the only way I knew to become someone important and to become a man.

When I was 16, I started my traineeship and started to train people. For many years I loved the fitness industry, and for the most part, I still do. Although around 19 something started to change for me. Something stopped making sense.

It was like in a single moment, everything I knew wasn't wrong; it was just incomplete.

I remember seeing one of the clients doing dumbbell bicep curls inches away from the mirror with headphones on and smashing down his fluorescent drink in between sets.

That moment is burned into my memory.

In that moment I had a thought: "This is not normal. Surely there is a better way to train."

In my late teens, but before this moment, I had made the connection that human beings are mammals. I know this is common knowledge; I am not claiming it. I am simply stating that I started to think if we are mammals/animals and we move and eat in particular ways, then why are we training in ways that go against human nature?

Now there are many answers to that question, and they are likely all correct yet incomplete.

For me everything changed from that moment. I stopped seeing going to the gym as a normal thing because for the greater part of human history it hasn't been.

It isn't normal to go to an air-conditioned facility, under fluorescent lights, run on electronic hamster wheels, and then break the body up into different parts to do robotic tedious movements that have no direct correlation to anything you do outside of that facility before shoving powders down your throat.

That's not to say that there aren't benefits to it; of course there are benefits. It just means that for a human mammal, this isn't a normal thing. It also isn't to say that I don't program bicep curls or make people use treadmills where necessary. Everything is contextual.

It just isn't normal.

Hell, flying in a plane isn't normal either, but it definitely has benefits.

The other thought that came up during this time in my life is, what other fallacies are hiding in the fitness industry?

Since that day in 2008, I have seen more and more of them come to life. Some are obvious, some are fads, and some are hidden right under our noses.

What I found was a large chunk of "professionals" or "influencers" marketing the beauty industry dressed up as the fitness industry and hidden in their sales scrips is a promise of an antidote to the low self-esteem that they are contributing to.

It's racketeering. They are solving the issues they themselves are creating.

Over time, the fitness industry moved away from being this ideal way to live a healthier life through weight training and jazzercize to a beauty industry preying on people's insecurities to make a buck.

A large part of the fitness industry creates and feeds long-term psychological issues and provides short-term physical solutions to create repeat customers.

This isn't to say that there aren't people within the fitness industry who genuinely care about the individuals they are communicating with and teaching because that would be a lie. There definitely are such people.

In today's climate there are a lot of people after a quick buck, and unfortunately that means a turnover of clients and often a turnover of results. If you are a trainer or a coach and you are on the fence between selling out or sticking with the truth and what is morally right, then stick to the truth. Keep telling the truth about the value of hard work and education. There is no eight-week challenge that can beat it. It will take time, but you will come out on top. Every community needs real leaders, not sellouts trying to flick a quick buck.

Now let me just reaffirm something here; this doesn't mean every single person who runs a challenge or sells an e-book. I am not saying never sign up to a newsletter or enter a challenge.

What I am saying is that there are people and businesses advocating a "healthy" lifestyle if you buy their product because you aren't good enough as you are or you are somehow inherently faulty.

That's bullshit.

And this book will show you why it is and how to move past that forever.

See what I did there.

There is a big difference though, and this is really important for you to understand.

That difference is *intention*.

My message isn't that you're not enough. My message is that you already are enough. You always have been. You just have to get rid of the crap that stands in your way and lies to your face.

So after training thousands of people and realizing that there is no one approach to health, fitness and happiness I have built a health map based on each individual's personal Health IQ.

It takes on board the physical approach to training and how that impacts the lives of people outside of the gym, as well as nutrition and being able to eat according to your goals and life conditions.

The big difference between the health map and your traditional diet and exercise programs is that I place a heavy emphasis on the mental game, a.k.a. mind-set.

Although I don't call it mind-set. Because I believe the mind should never be set. Like health and human beings as a whole, your mind is constantly shifting, adapting, expanding.

In fact, it could be argued that mind-*set* is one of the issues.

Some of us are walking around with our minds set from our teenage years, and it is heavily impacting how we show up today as adults

Time to free your mind, not set it.

Let me give you an example of how the mind can heavily impact the rest of our health.

Let's say we have a female who, when she was in high school, was bullied for being slightly larger and heavier than "the skinny bitches." She was comforted by her mum and told that the whole family is heavyset, and those girls are unhappy and lashing out at her because she is happy, those damn "skinny bitches." Let's also say that this female really values happiness, and as she gets older and she continues to slowly get heavier she comes to the realization in her 30s that she wants to lose weight. Consciously she works toward her goal, going to the gym, eating "healthy" food, and even going as far as getting a personal trainer. She starts to lose a bit of weight and things are moving in the right direction. She continues to lose more, and kilo by kilo it starts to slow down.

And so does her attention to detail in regard to healthy eating and her training sessions. Before she knows it, she is pretty much back to her starting weight a few short months after things "got busy."

She does this a couple of times throughout her thirties. Now she's in her forties, and she's trying again, but this time she also has a track record of how many times she's failed to lose weight in the past. So she feels that no matter what she does, she'll always self-sabotage her goal of losing weight. This leads her to think that she's a failure and that she's simply just not a "healthy person." She starts to believe that exercise and dieting make her unhappy, which therefore makes her unhealthy. What we may be forgiven for missing here is the fact that she may hold a higher frame (another word for "belief") that if she were to lose weight, she would become a skinny bitch, and she will become unhappy. So unbeknown to her she has this belief back in her subconscious that is appearing to be sabotaging her goals. Every time she gets close to achieving a goal, she pulls away and "fails" because she values happiness, and she connects being a skinny bitch to being unhappy.

There isn't a diet in the world that can help somebody overcome this without addressing underlying causes that their frames and beliefs may be contributing to.

Some people's hard work isn't in the gym; it isn't in the kitchen or the supermarket. It is in the mind. It is going in and understanding what frames we hold in mind that are governing the games in life.

Remember this: the highest frame (think belief) governs the game.

People often think they self-sabotage, but they don't. Often their conscious goals are simply in conflict with their unconscious beliefs. What this means for people in this situation is that if they were to actually achieve their conscious goal it would be sabotaging their unconscious beliefs. We act in accordance to our unconscious beliefs.

Without truly understanding this, you can leave people to thinking that there's something wrong with them, that they are inherently faulty, and that they are always going to be a failure. There is simply more to health than what meets the eye. Hence my point that there is more to health than diet and exercise.

This isn't to say that mind-set is everything, because it's not everything. Your mind, your movement, and your food are all integrated.

Health is a continual dance of movement, mindset, and what goes into our mouths.

What Even Is Health?

Minding yourself is about being more human in a world that profits from our insecurities, laziness, and low self-esteem. It is about learning what you need to do in order to live your best life. It is about looking after yourself first so that you can lead others. It is about learning to understand our own minds so that we can clear the crap and live up to our potential.

At the core, it's about being human.

Being "human" can look different for each and every individual, and there is a significant amount of differences depending on what this can look like and feel like for you. One of the most important things to truly understand is that health is not something static. It is a dynamic process.

Health is forever unfolding and continually shifting.

What worked for you when you were 20 probably won't work for you when you are 30 and most likely won't work for you when you are 40. Not just from a physical standpoint but also from a priority standpoint, financial standpoint, mental standpoint, and there are many, many other factors that can come into play, such as family and career change.

So in the process of understanding this, it is very important to also grasp that this isn't a 12-week challenge or a fat-loss program. This is a continually unfolding and evolving process, which is exactly what you are. You are not a snapshot in time. You are not an Instagram post. You are continually unravelling and evolving. Because of this, this book will recommend small changes daily that, when built upon over a year, can begin to drastically revolutionize your life.

The truth of the matter is that we cannot get healthy in 12 weeks. We can get fitter, we can lose weight, but we cannot become healthy in 12 weeks.

Let me explain why: health is a continually lived state that incorporates and integrates all areas of our lives.

Here are some examples of what health is *not*:

- Body composition
- A number on the scales

- What someone else thinks of you
- Your current diet regime
- A six-pack
- An Instagram post
- A gym membership
- A personal trainer

It is integral to understand that health is not any one individual thing but rather a continual dynamic pull among the many facets of our lives that we have control or influence of. Some of these are subjective like our thoughts and our community support, and some others are objective like our body and the location where we exercise.

Following is a list of examples of some of the factors that contribute to good health:

- The people we spend time with
- Being true to our own truth and speaking our truth
- Moving our body in a way that empowers us
- Food that grows from the ground or had a mum
- The environments we decide to spend our time in
- Being conscious and aware of our thoughts
- Taking complete responsibility for what is within our power
- Letting go of things, thoughts, and situations that no longer serve us
- Being present (like actually present, being here, now, as you are, in this moment, no bullshit, no spiritual materialism, just fully here)

Over the years, I have seen many people sacrifice progress for results. It is "The Tortoise and the Hare" story. They say that life is short, and as true as that is, life is also the longest thing you will ever do. Play the long game when it comes to your health. The short game can be both financially expensive and also emotionally expensive. Keep focused on what truly matters for you and make sure your health enables you to do exactly that.

One of the higher frames I like to keep and offer to those who are inclined that way is that it is far healthier to have a beer or wine with some friends and a good laugh than it is to bitch about people while eating a salad.

Salad doesn't unbitch you.

Once again, health is so much more than the food we eat and the way we move.

And as we know, too much beer and wine brings its own problems. More on that later.

The Only Two Things That Matter

One of the biggest influences on the way that I coach and educate came from a very powerful lesson I learned when attending a very dear friend's funeral back in December 2016. I am not sure you can really prepare yourself to walk your best friend to their hearse. I know I sure as hell wasn't prepared. During Alex's funeral, it occurred to me that there really are only two things in life that matter; everything else is just noise. Everything else is just a distraction.

Those two things are as follows:

1. How you contribute
2. The memories you make

Alex was 28 when he had his car accident. There were no witnesses, and it involved two cars travelling in opposite directions.

At his funeral no one spoke about his couch or his house. They didn't speak about his bank account or the amount of likes he got on his posts. They didn't talk about how much he weighed or what he could lift. They didn't talk about how he came fifth in some weekend competition.

They only talked about those two things.

Alex was both a teacher and a videographer, and those who shared stories about him spoke about how he was always the first person on set to give a hand, moving things, and how he was always the last to leave. They talked about the social work he did that next to no one knew about. They talked about the memories they had of him and how he contributed to not just their lives but the community as a whole.

They talked about what mattered. Everything else would have been just be a distraction.

There was another time I was sitting down and talking to one of the dads who trains at my gym. He had just finished his session and was talking to me about how he was frustrated about not getting stronger. I get that, sure; the issue here was that his reference point was another guy from another gym at a weekend competition. I asked him why that mattered in the long run and also reminded him that what does matter is teaching his son how to bench press in their garage gym when his son was 16. He didn't need to get stronger; he needed to refocus on what was important and train for that. You can replace just about anything with "bench press." Playing catch, going fishing, whatever. The point is that his focus shifted from what matters long term to what matters short term.

I am deeply ingrained to the philosophy that you should train to build memories and live to contribute to a cause bigger than yourself.

Regret is a rough teacher. It only hands us the answers to the lessons long after the opportunity to do anything about them has gone. It is said that the best time to plant a tree is 20 years ago and the second-best time is now. The same thing can be said for taking the necessary steps to take control of our health. No matter where you are at in your life, you have the ability to stave off regret by doing small things today that lead you to living your best life.

I have seen people turn their lives around at 60 because they had a brand-new addition in the family, which crowned them a grandparent. They made the decision to make sure that they were remembered for being the grandparent who was still active and still playful.

We can often get caught up in the pursuit of trivial shit when it comes to life and our health. The truth is that no one cares what you weigh. No one cares how much you lift. No one cares about your social media likes. Your kids? They will remember you for how you participated in life with them. How you contributed to their development and growth. They don't care what you weigh on the scales. They want you to be happy, not to yo-yo. Your friends (unless you have shitty friends who make you unhappy or hold you back) want to see you genuinely happy and not faking it because fake happiness is the worst type of sadness.

The truth is no one wants to lose weight.

Seriously, hear me out.

Firstly, no one wants to lose. Most, if not all, of us grew up knowing the difference between a winner and a loser, between winning and losing. Generally speaking, winning = good, losing = bad. I mean what is the point of putting in all this hard work just to lose.

Buried deep in so many people's unconscious is a negative connotation to losing, and it totally makes sense. Of course, not everyone is exactly the same, I am talking about a general meme within the greater society: however traditionally people want to win, they want to gain something, and, ironically, to become more of something, sometimes we have to lose something. The funny thing is that whenever we lose, we also gain, and whenever we win, we also lose. You cannot have one without the other. If you lose weight you may gain confidence. If you lose friends, you may feel a sense of new freedom you didn't think you had when they were around. When we let go of and lose old beliefs, we gain the ability to choose new, powerful frames that can help govern us to a new way of living that is best aligned with unravelling our potential.

Secondly, it isn't weight loss people are after anyway. It is what they think they will gain from weight loss. So potentially confidence, attractiveness, freedom from pain, freedom to play with their children and not be seen to be the lazy parent who was too unhealthy to play with them (maybe because that's what their parents were in their eyes). So if it is not weight loss that you want, what is it? Maybe the goal isn't weight loss, maybe it is strength, toning, fitness, to be pain free, to lift a certain amount, run a certain distance. No matter what it is, why do you want that? Why is it important to you? What do you think achieving that will give you that you don't already have? You see, it is a complex topic. So many people lose weight and feel elated for a short period of time. The get the before and after photos out, maybe a few hundred likes on the socials, and some really nice externally validating comments. They get the high that comes with all that. But somewhere after a few days, it starts to go away. It starts to just dissipate into thin air, hoping that maybe someone might comment on the photo again so it pops back up in newsfeeds and people who didn't like it the first time will get the opportunity to like it again. It's like happiness is the cake, but the cake is almost gone, and all is to pick up the crumbs. And so we do, until there are no crumbs left.

Time to go make another cake, hey?

The truth is in order to have long-term health it is worth going deep within our own minds and being honest with ourselves as to why we may want what we want. Is it to prove someone wrong? Is it to finally get our parents validation or approval? Is it to continue to be seen in the eyes of our peers as a high achiever? Is it because no matter how much I achieve, I always feel empty, but I just don't know how to live any other way, so I continue to achieve things so that I can have the fleeting moments of high that come with achieving even if no one else finds out about it? Does that cause me to never be at rest but always feel like there is pressure to tick off the next thing on my list that never seems to stop growing because "it just who I am"?

That is why it is worth asking ourselves, what do we really want? After I remove all of the justifying and the superficial white lies I tell myself, what do I really want?

We are meaning-making machines, and we have all made a meaning about what healthy means to us.

What does it mean to you?

One thing I know for sure is that what does make us healthy are not just the improvements in fitness and fat loss but how we think, how we make meaning of the world, and the complete ownership of what is within our control.

It is so important to understand that life happens for us, not to us. One way to think about this is when something challenging happens in our life. Do we tell ourselves that this bad thing happened to us? Or did this challenging situation happen for us so we can grow and become who we truly deserve to be?

We get to choose how we want to participate, and you don't build memories from the sidelines.

I have written this book to challenge you in so many different ways. From the way you currently think (or think you think) to the way we move, exercise, eat, and interact with those around us.

Throughout the book we will cover all this and more as we navigate what truly is important to you and what mental strategies, physical training, and nutrition plans can look like to support your life and goals out there in the real world.

There is only one catch: this book can't do the work for you. I can't do the work for you. Your spouse can't do the work for you. The work is up to you. You have to earn it by doing the process and over time falling in love with the process rather than forcing yourself to do things you hate for some hopeful pay off in a few months' time.

Since 2004 I have been fortunate enough to train somewhere over 5,000 people and have done a lot of the hard work for you. I have learned the common patterns people fall into that will cause them to yo-yo. I have heard the difference in the language of those who are successful at their goals and those who fall short—again and again. I have learned that what you gain quickly, you lose quickly. I have learned that your body is the only place you have to live for your whole life, so it is best to spend the time taking care of it than to try and make "renovations" (or worse, a knock down rebuild) later in life.

So, after all of that, if you are ready, it is time to start Minding YourSELF.

Who Is This Book For?

Minding yourSELF is for any person who wants to look past the typical diet and gym world and step into a deeper understanding of themselves and their subjective experience of how they think and then integrate that with their physical world of diet and exercise.

One of the key factors in long-term success is being ready to make a change. As cliché as it sounds, leading a horse to water is one thing. This book is the water; the practices that are offered throughout it are an opportunity for you to drink. I can't make you do that.

The horse will only drink if it is thirsty.

So the question is, are you thirsty? Are you ready?

If you are, then it is important that we talk about what it will cost you.

I am not talking financial although financial is important for a couple of reasons. One being the fact that when people pay, they pay attention, and another being that what we invest in our ourselves has a direct correlation to what we believe we are worth. The important thing to understand with that though is that an investment can be monetary; it could be charitable or even an investment of time. There are many different ways to invest in ourselves, but don't be fooled, there is a direct correlation to self-worth.

The most important cost to discuss is that a transition into a new life or way of seeing the world will cost you your old. It may cost you some friends, maybe some family, maybe some money, but definitely your old frames (beliefs), habits, and behaviors. The good news is that it also means the old suffering and pain you have either undergone in silence or maybe in a more public setting can also be cleared.

If that is what you want.

One of the early pioneers of the Enneagram (which you will learn about later), George Gurdjieff, is quoted saying that the last thing people will let go of is their suffering.

Why?

Because it is so entangled with and fused into their identity, their significance, and their story. If you were to take away their suffering, then what would make them feel important? What would make them feel worthy of being heard? What would justify their behaviors and story if they were to be freed from their suffering?

The truth is a lot of people don't want to let go of that. And it makes complete sense. It is brave to let go of the things that explain why we aren't worthy or good enough or strong enough. It makes sense why we then look for this externally in other people, achievements, or parental figures.

So the key thing is, are you able to identify what you want to let go of in order to move into a higher level of being for yourself. If so, you are going to have to be okay with being wrong. With being fallible, with being human.

Because the thinking that got you to where you are won't get you to where you want to go.

Like a snake, there comes a time to shed that old skin.

A time when for us all, holding onto things that no longer serve us becomes more painful than letting them go.

So how do we get to that point? Well, that is a complicated topic once again. One thing that is for sure is that this can and will be different for each individual person. Something that is crucial to outline is that when the student is ready, the teacher will appear, and that won't be because the teacher wasn't there. The teacher was always there; the student first had to develop the curiosity and recognize the possibility that there is a different way of perceiving the world before they could seek out a teacher.

The teacher is always there and especially now more than ever. With books, podcasts, webinars, video calls, and so much information at our fingertips it is both so easy to be the student and seek out teachers and also to be the know it all and get stuck in ignorance and reductionist views.

Never forget that curiosity keeps us young and ignorance ages our soul.

Life Conditions

I read once that comparison is the thief of joy, and in today's climate, it is easier than ever to compare ourselves to someone or something external to ourselves.

Couple that comparison with the pressure we put on ourselves to perform to a high standard in our life, whether that be at work, in our community, as a mother, or at school or in all these areas, and it makes complete sense that we can become our biggest critic.

One of the most crucial things for us to do is to be honest with ourselves about the priority of using the gym, sticking to our diet, and training when it comes to our current life conditions.

There are times in our lives where we can really put the foot down on the accelerator on our health or the gym or training for an event, and there are times where we can pull back. Where people can go wrong with this is when they see it as an either/or situation.

Our health is not an either/or situation. It is a relationship, and like any other long-term successful relationship we must calibrate and prioritize different things at different times. Hence one of the issues—being on a diet or falling off the bandwagon. There is no bandwagon; there is no diet. There is only food, education, and priorities. We may become more focused and measured with what we eat, but we are always eating. Therefore we always have "a diet" so to speak.

The importance of being able to take life conditions into account is that it actually allows us to not take on too much or to end up "falling off the wagon." We start to see our training, development, and nutrition more like a dimmer than simply a switch. We can turn it up and turn it down when it suits the situation.

One key thing to understand is that training isn't always exercise. Although I will expand on this much later in the movement component of this book, what I want to point out here is that if we are not getting enough recovery and sleep, let's say it is because work has gotten busier and the kids aren't sleeping well, which is impacting our sleep, then it is normal to end up feeling more stressed as a result of all this. A common desire might be to "push through" and smash out the gym to relieve stress. Hey, I am all for pushing through difficult periods. But I am not all for doing it by sacrificing your long-term health. If we are stressed at work and we are stressed at home and then stressing ourselves to go to the gym, then going to the gym and smashing out a workout is more stress on the body!

My point here is that there are times where pulling back the intensity or the amount of time spent at the gym may be beneficial for you in the long term rather than simply just pushing through, getting less sleep, and feeling more and more stressed overall.

Once again, another factor to take into account with our health is our current life condition.

Why is this important? Well one reason is that it feeds into when people are ready or not. As much as I am an advocate for radical self-responsibility, there are still times where things out of your control will impact your day-to-day life, and the only thing you can control (as challenging as it is sometimes) is your response to the situation.

The other reason is that our awareness of this principle can help build sensory acuity with what is required of us in any given moment. Without this, we can become blind to old rules and principles that may fall into an all-or-nothing paradigm, and even though they may have served us at some point in our life, if we lack flexibility in the moment, then nothing serves us.

One of the traits of people who are extremely successful in this area is their capability for behavioral adaptability. This is not to be confused with changing our personality to gain approval or to manipulate someone. Behavioral adaptability is one's ability to adapt to any given circumstances based on what is required in that moment in one's life. This can be governed by overarching personal values, frames/beliefs, and principles; however, it gives one flexibility and freedom in the moment to have those things and not be had by them.

There is a massive difference between being had by our values and frames and us having them. Carl Jung had a quote that fed into this ideology, which said,

"Do people have ideas or do ideas have people?"

Have your goals, have your beliefs, have your values and principles. Just don't be had by them. To truly lean into your potential, you must learn to be flexible in the moment and not rigidly adhere to an outdated personal doctrine.

How to Deal With Friends and Family When Going Through Change

Our sensory acuity of our own life conditions is crucial. Our awareness that other people have their own life conditions is also really important.

For a long time, I struggled with the concept of someone's "journey." It felt too cliché or lacking substance until I realized that each and every person is going through their own unfolding. As some mature and develop and make decisions, others are unravelling at different times. The unravelling is our journey. I have one and so do you, whether you're conscious of it or not.

So this next stage, the next development you undergo, is really twofold. Firstly, how do I make sure I am supported, and how do I support other people on their journey?

Dealing with friends and family when going through a growth transition is multifaceted. There is the part where they either support us or don't and then there is the part where we may want to project our goals and newfound knowledge onto them. These can both be very challenging topics to dance around and, if left unaddressed, they can really impact our home life and our happiness.

Although it is nice and all warm and fuzzy when you are supported by friends and family, the simple truth is that what is more important than them supporting you and believing you is you supporting yourself and believing in yourself. People believing in you doesn't mean shit if you don't believe in yourself. The reason is because you can only treat someone as good as they treat themselves. So often the question isn't, how do people treat me? It is, how do I treat myself?

So if you don't already treat yourself well, it may be worth considering that you are worth taking care of. Because you are.

This isn't to rule out the importance of having a support group. This is to point out the importance of both the support from others and, most importantly, the support from yourself. A lot of people may struggle for self-worth, so they look for it in other people's words and actions. This type of conditional self-worth is common, but it doesn't have to be normal. One of the keys to true success is building unwavering self-belief. This may take time and it may feel silly in the beginning, but stick with it, and, in the long run, you will take your power back and in turn give more of yourself back to the world than you ever could have if you were still searching for your self-worth in other people.

So step one is to support yourself. Why would we expect other people to support us if we don't support ourselves? That's not to say they won't; it's just putting the onus on us to take responsibility.

Are You Actually Helping?

During this unravelling and your personal development, you will attain some amazing new insights and knowledge that you may want to share with those around you.

My advice is to tread carefully.

There is a quote that I remember by Alan Watts, and it spoke profoundly to me as a trainer and coach.

"Please let me help save you or you will drown, said the Monkey to the Fish, putting it up a tree."

Sometimes it can be so easy to see the solutions to other people's problems and offer advice, especially when it hasn't been sought. But often, we may be looking at a singular problem being either voiced by them or maybe it hasn't been voiced by them but rather just observed by us, through our eyes and not theirs.

So we want to jump in and help them with all this new information and knowledge and, of course, our love.

There are four interesting factors about this type of situation.

Firstly, did the person ask for our advice, or did we prequalify that they wanted it? I can think of numerous times where I have been on both sides of this: giving unsolicited advice without prequalifying it and then complaining about people not taking it on board or brushing me off. I can also empathize with them as people have projected their advice onto me to "fix" my "problem" without fully understanding it or prequalifying that I actually want their input, only for them to get upset when I told them to stop. In all fairness, I know I have the talent to be blunt, so when letting them know I was not interested in their "chunks of wisdom," I may have left out a few please and thank-yous.

My strong connection to the traits of a type 8 on the Enneagram may help to explain this more. But more on that in the mind part of the book.

So in short, ask if the person would like your input before just dishing out your turd sandwich. Remember that most of the time, we are simply making the turd sandwich as best we can, from the resources and ingredients we have. And sometimes, it is shit.

Even if it is a delicious sandwich, if they didn't order it, they probably don't want it or they at least won't respect it.

Anyhow, secondly, are we simply projecting our own values onto others without taking into account their life conditions and also our own blind spots? It is a challenging question because we are often coming from a place of love and care. It's just that we may not truly be listening to them and understanding what's important to them but rather projecting what's important to us.

Are we projecting what we value onto them and assuming they either do or should value the same thing? Are we advising on their situation based off our values? Do we have a bias in the situation? Does the other person? Do I have a desire to look supportive and be the "nice guy/girl," to be seen as always helpful and always reliable? To always have the answer?

Often the people who help the most need the most help. They don't know how to "fix" their life, so they go about trying to fix everyone else's. One hundred percent of the feel-goods and 0 percent of the responsibility. A lot of the time being helpful is really unhelpful, and for a number of reasons, one of them being that sometimes we struggle seeing other people in pain (which is the pain of seeing other people struggle), and so we jump in and try and get rid of their pain. Which, inadvertently, is an attempt to rid ourselves of our discomfort and most likely an attempt to uphold an external image to other people. But who are we to know that they don't need this struggle? There is the metaphor that when you help a butterfly out of a cocoon, out of its struggle, you not only weaken it, but you also impair its ability to fly. This makes it codependent upon a carer, which, in turn, can uphold the carer's identity as an empath who cares for such poor souls. This, by the way, is noble, as long as we aren't the thing that made them codependent or are the reason they stay codependent.

More on co-dependencies later. For now, my offer is to become acutely aware as to whether you are projecting your values upon other people, which is aiding a bias in your advice. It's a tough pill to swallow yet so transformational for all parties.

The third one is, do they even want to get rid of their suffering? I refer to George Gurdjieff's quote earlier that some people don't want to end their suffering. The fact that people (maybe you are on either end of this equation) keep giving them attention because of it can often make them feel important. Of course, so much of this is occurring unconsciously and is simply feeding deeper needs such as significance, protection/safety, and love. That aside, my offer for you is to focus on your stuff, to be an example, and, where possible, lead people to their own conclusions rather than instill your values upon them. This can be ironic because throughout this book I am offering different views, different bits of advice, and also potentially new ideas. That's why you will often hear me (or read me) saying "Here is an offer." I am assuming that you have picked up this book and are reading it because you are wanting to learn more and are seeking out different ways to do things. My deepest offer is that whatever you take from this book, own it. Own all of it. Take full responsibility for your decisions and frames of reference moving forward. When we do that, it is powerful, and that is how we empower ourselves.

The fourth and final point to be made from this situation is, do we understand the whole problem space? Do others even understand the whole problem space? What even is a problem space? Allow me to explain: a problem space is seeing the whole picture and asking questions that the individual experiencing the problem may have not even thought of yet. Often we can get to advising from hearing the problem but without understanding the problem space. The problem may exist in one area, yet the problem space can stretch over many other areas of that person's life.

Let's use the losing weight example again. Someone wants to lose weight. That's pretty simple; here is their problem: they weigh more than they want to. So they want to weigh less. Okay, here is a diet and an exercise regime and off you go.

Doesn't work. They don't get their desired result.

So we start to hear comments like the person must not have stuck to it. They mustn't be motivated. They must be undisciplined and lazy. They just don't want it. They aren't ready. They aren't committed.

Possibly, or maybe we haven't been able to figure out the problem space. Let's say their partner, whom they love dearly, struggles with their own self-worth and is overweight themselves. Their partner is at their own stage of unfolding within their own life conditions. This particular partner starts to project their insecurities onto their beloved partner, who is trying to lose weight.

"Just have the cake, hunny." "You're beautiful as you are." "You're not overweight." "You're not spending enough times with the kids." "Why are you spending so much money on that health stuff?" "We just aren't like that; we aren't the fitness types." And so on, and so on.

So this person is in fear that if they lose weight, they will lose the person they love. And if they lose the person they love, they will lose access to their kids, and they will be less worthy and be miserable.

All this is operating in the background.

But, hey, they're just lazy right?

So how do we get this person to lose weight?

A lot of people won't like my answer.

You don't.

They have to come to that conclusion and seek the answer to the questions when they are ready. Maybe they aren't breaking out of the cocoon yet, or maybe they are starting to. Let them go through the challenge. It will allow them to come to the solution themselves and start to own it. They will become stronger and wiser from their struggle. When you take on their struggle, you often weaken them, and when they start to own it, they start to achieve it. It becomes something they no longer need to be motivated for; it is a part of who they are.

This is where real long-term change happens.

Now we can always influence people, but once again, the horse must be thirsty.

One of the key reasons I am sharing these four principles to be aware of when it comes to attempting to motivate or influence someone else is to allow you insight that although you may go through some serious changes throughout the course of this book and beyond, other people may not. And, my offer for you would be to become okay with that. Everyone is unfolding at their own pace just as you are. The second reason is that maybe the examples feel close to home, maybe your spouse, your parent, friend, or other family member. More importantly, maybe you can relate to the examples given.

Either way, the important thing is to become okay with the process of everything unfolding as it is. Especially when it comes to yourself.

You are not meant to be anywhere else at this point in your life.

You were not meant be to already fit, skinny, at a particular weight, or anything. In fact, that type of thinking usually keeps us unfit, overweight, and unhappy.

I will quite often refer to the universe unfolding as it is and to focus on what is within your control and become aware of what truly does make you happy, to also be able to see previous conditions you placed on your self-worth and confidence, your happiness, and your love.

People can sometimes get caught up in wanting things to happen faster. That is literally like sitting in the middle of the river and using your arms to try and make the river move faster.

You cannot make the river move faster.

You can only unblock the things in its way so that it moves at the rate it is capable of. Clear the rocks so the river can flow.

Clear the crap.

When we see the things in the way of our potential, we can learn to accept them, move through them, integrate them, and allow the universe to continue to unfold (just like the river) as it always has without our personal judgment of how we specifically think reality and the universe should be.

This is what it means to get out of our own way.

Most fitness books won't talk about it, because they don't know how to. They don't know how to talk about the work of getting out of our own way.

As well as movement and nutrition, we will also be discussing how to identify the patterns we have created that has slowed down the flow of our river. Then, how to identify the rocks in order to allow our river to flow freely again.

To recap these points, below are some questions worth considering.

1. Do they/I truly want to get rid of their suffering? If this suffering could have a positive intention, what could that be?
2. Am I simply projecting my own values onto someone else?
3. Have I asked questions truly wanting to understand their/my problem space?
4. Has the person even asked for feedback? Did I ask if they would like my feedback? Did I simply provide it without qualifying if they wanted it or not?

How Do You Know You Are Ready?

The fact that you're reading this book is a pretty good sign that you are ready for the next stage. We are all at different stages of development be that in our work life, our relationships, or our health.

The question is, if you are physically healthy, but you hate your job and you fight with your spouse often, then just how healthy are you?

Are you healthier than someone who absolutely loves their work, spends copious amounts of time with their children, and has a balanced and open communicative relationship with their significant other?

Who is healthier?

The fact is, health just looks different on each person. This is why it is so important to identify what health means to us. As challenging as it is, health isn't just about expanding our strengths, which, in the examples above, would be the physical body for the first person and relationships and loving their job for the second. Health is also about looking at the parts of us we don't like. The parts of us that we may have rejected. Health is a constant pursuit of our potential, and our potential lies in broadening our awareness rather than just doubling down on strengths.

This is why this book is designed in a way to challenge you. It will challenge you to go to places that maybe you have resisted for some time. To have a look at old beliefs and frames that you didn't even know that you had. To try some new types of physical training. To up level your nutrition so that you can up level your life.

So if you aren't ready to be challenged, then this book isn't for you.

If you are ready to be challenged and are ready to let go of the crap that has held you, then it's clear, you are ready.

As mentioned earlier, there is one thing that is certain. No one else can do the work for you. A lot of the personal trainers and coaches I work with struggle with this. They feel overly responsible for their clients' results and take it personally. If a client doesn't get the result that they want, they almost feel like it is an attack on their own integrity and identity. It's not; the person will get the result when they are ready.

I am not responsible for my clients' results.

They are.

Just like you.

If I take responsibility for their results, then I also take responsibility for their failures. If I accept their wins, then I also learn their lessons, and that's just plain not fair. I end up weakening them, not empowering them. I played a role, just like the next person, but I didn't make you pick up this book. I didn't make you read this line. You chose to do that, or not to do it, and at any point, if you are not up to the challenge, then you're welcome to opt out. No judgment. Because not everyone is ready for the work.

The truth about the work though is that it is small steps. Small continuous steps. No matter where you are at in your life. People will walk into the gym and proclaim that they have so many things to work on. They have the same number of things as me.

One thing. That's all. The next thing. Whatever that may be for them. One of the best rules that you can bring to secure your long-term development is don't practice something until you get it right; practice until you can't get it wrong.

So if you ever get overwhelmed, it is probably because you are looking too far ahead and not doing anything now. Breathe and ask yourself, what is the one thing that is in my power that I can do right now and get to actioning it? The overwhelm goes away with this action.

This is true motivation.

Motivation means to move toward action. It's not just sitting on the couch and some sort of magical wave of motivation hitting us (and if it does, it is usually extrinsic/external motivation—be careful) and then we get up and go crush our goals. No, we are on the couch, but by taking action we become motivated. That is a really, really important distinction.

The other important distinction is that if you have to be motivated to do something, don't worry about it. It isn't important to you. If motivation happens while doing something that is important to you, then great! Otherwise, if it is important to you, you won't need it. You will just go about getting it done.

So the key thing is to understand that you actually don't need motivation to achieve what you want. Motivation is what happens when you have already taken action toward what you want. Most people aren't lazy; they just have uninspiring goals and targets to move toward. They don't have something that is compelling enough to move toward and something painful enough to move away from. Having both allows us to have a healthy push-pull toward a worthy ideal. A push away from pain and a pull toward a compelling future.

We build a home by placing one brick at a time. We do the same with our lives.

Throughout this book, I have offers for you that will allow you to take one step at a time, learn it, develop it, and then integrate it into your lifestyle.

So if you are ready to take the next step for you, your next step is defining what you want and where you want to go.

After that, you will learn where you are placed on the Health IQ Map and then where you need to be in order to achieve the goal you wish to. The Health IQ Map will point you to the steps you can take to get to where you want to be.

But first, let's take a deeper look at the fitness industry, marketing, and the media.

Consciously Wire Your Unconscious

There are some themes in this book that may appear to either repeat themselves or overlap. This has been done on purpose to show how much all the topics and examples in this book are interconnected. I once heard the quote "repetition is the mother of all skill," and this has governed so much of my learning since.

If we want to get better at something or develop a skill, we repeat it. Our unconscious mind is constantly working and picking information up. Although the numbers vary slightly from study to study, we process up to eleven million bits of information a second, yet our conscious mind is only observant of about fifty. This is why we know words to songs we don't even like, we recall bits of information we didn't realize we had, and we forget things that we only read or hear once.

Often I hear people say they don't read because they cannot retain the information they do read. If you can read and you don't retain what you read, then it is as good as not being able to read. There is an African proverb that reads, "When a man dies, a library burns to the ground." I urge you to take notes throughout this book, follow up on the links and other reading materials. Use this book as a resource for further your study. I am not telling you what to see; I am pointing you where to look. What you see is up to you.

My other offer is that if something piques your interest, follow it. If something in this book brings up something in you, whether that be the training component, the nutrition component, or even a throwaway passage, my offer and recommendation is to pursue it. Google it and also have a look at my recommended reading list that you can find at www.davenixon.com.au.

Whatever you do keep studying.

When we hear the same thing a few times, we can start to better understand it rather than it just remaining information. The more we hear something or read something or study something, we have the opportunity to truly start pulling apart its meaning and its intention.

There is a quote by an ancient Greek philosopher named Heraclitus that says, "No man ever steps in the same river twice, for it's not the same river and he's not the same man."

When you come across something in life, you can understand it only up to the level that your life experience, education, and maturity will allow you to at that point. The more you come across it as you move through life, the deeper you can connect with it. The deeper connection we have with ourselves, the deeper connection we have with what we come across.

Sometimes this can be lost as some wishy-washy feel-good stuff, and that is the exact lie that prevents us from building a true connection with ourselves and the world.

The main thing I point out in this book is our internal world. We will cover food and exercise and all the actionable objective content, but we cannot move forward personally or globally if we don't look within and understand that person there.

A lot of people have a high level of emotional intelligence when it comes to other people but lack it when it comes to themselves. The interesting thing is that it is called emotional IN-telligence, not OUT-telligence. To be emotionally illiterate, we must go in.

This is my INvitation for you.

The Health of the Fitness Industry

The fitness industry is sick. I know I have talked a bit about it already, but it is important for our own health that we dig a little deeper and make some serious distinctions about it.

If we aren't careful, we can get taken down a very shiny and well-marketed alleyway by an extremely fit presenting individual to purchase a load of unnecessary supplements and pursue other people's goals that hold the promise of a happier life.

I actually love the fitness and health industry. I do. It gave me the opportunity to do what I do and to learn, to meet some amazing people and learn some really tough lessons. I have also learned how much of the industry isn't what it says it is.

The reality is that there are a lot of people walking around with one title while they really are acting in a different way.

Marketing has become a dangerous thing within the fitness industry. Unfortunately, a lot of the advice you see about sales and marketing is simple: point at (or create) a problem someone has and then show how your product or service will fix it. Make sure to explain that it won't only fix it, but will fix it like nothing else ever possibly could. Tell them (you) it is better, superior, and easier than all the rest.

Too many entry-level personal trainers and instructors have spent more time with their heads in marketing books and listening to YouTube videos of fitness marketers than being personally invested in the client in front of them. They are distracting themselves with what really matters. That is doing the years on the floor with the clients and learning and learning and learning. It is as if they don't want to fail. It is like they don't want to look stupid or be seen as stupid in a world that is full of 60-second video clips into another person's life that is only interrupted by a perfectly angled and filtered photo. That's just not real.

And that is where we as an industry fall short. We promise too much and deliver too little. We take complex problems and simplify them. We become overly responsible for our clients' results so that we look good. We run challenges and take before and after photos and tell everyone how good we are because, "look at these results." Our clients achieved them because of us, but it is the clients' fault they lost them.

You have people walking around as personal trainers who at their core are simply marketers. You have people self-proclaiming their fitness influence status when the only thing they care about is influencing their bank account through endorsements.

There is a difference between a marketer in the fitness industry and a personal trainer learning how to market.

Of course, this isn't everyone in the industry. It may not even be the majority. But it is the loud minority.

It is really important to point out that I am not against commercial facilities, marketing, sales, supplements, or diet programs and especially not those that give out business advice on social media. My word of warning is to do your homework. Be responsible for your health and be responsible for where you get your education from.

A part of the industry is also just outright lies. They promote products, diets, or training programs to get the body that you want while promoting these with the body *they* have. The issue lies in how many people are not disclosing the truth, and, honestly, it is really hard to tell who is being honest and who isn't.

Say, for example, you have a female fitness influencer who is promoting the whole fitness package for aspiring females. The package includes a diet, a number of supplements, and a training program. They promote it with pictures of themselves in bikinis, which have them carefully positioned, light edited, and professionally taken. What they are selling here isn't a celebration of what the body can do; it is selling what the body can look like. In short, they are inadvertently saying that if you take these supplements, eat according to my diet template, and follow my program, then you too can have this body.

What could this mean? That you aren't good enough without looking like this? That if you look like this then you will be worthy of love? That the fact you don't look like this is why you're not happy? Can it be encouraging conditional esteem and happiness? Overvaluing a physical image over mental health? It is hard to say. It will vary for each individual.

What we don't see is any cosmetic work that the influencer has done. From breast augmentation to Botox to butt lifts. We don't see the supplements or the performance enhancing drugs (PEDs) that they are possibly taking without our knowledge. We really don't see anything that they don't want to show us.

What harm can this do? Well, take one of the aspiring fitness warriors purchasing the program; she may want to feel good about herself, look and feel more attractive, and be comfortable in her own skin. She may already have conditional self-esteem (always think of "esteem" as another word for "worth") and self-confidence. So she buys the program, follows it to the letter, and no matter how hard she tries, she never looks like the girl in the photos promoting it. "What's wrong with me?" she questions.

Nothing, sweetheart. Nothing is wrong with you. They tricked you into thinking something was. There never has been.

"The girl in the magazine doesn't even look like the girl in the magazine."

This is not just unique to women. It is universal.

Let's flip the script. Let's say someone is ready to make a change, and this is where they start. Is that so bad? What happens if it wasn't for this person marketing what they were marketing and the aspiring individual who bought the program came across it at the exact time she decided to make a change? Maybe she didn't achieve the long-term change advertised in this program, but over the next couple of years she continued to educate herself and make some serious long-term change. Is it so bad now?

You see, it is complex. There are many factors that go into the whole situation. One thing is for sure, if you want long-term change, you will get it. You will hunt down how to do it, and you will make it happen. If you aren't ready, then you won't, and maybe that's because there isn't enough pain pushing you to changing yet, you don't know what to move forward to, or you don't think you deserve it. There could be a whole heap of reasons.

It does go without saying that my description above does not fit every single fitness trainer with an Instagram. There are thousands who are really honest and up-front. They promote products and services they believe in and use themselves. They have the integrity to only promote what they do and are transparent. If you are in the fitness industry as a coach, trainer, or instructor then please, keep speaking the truth. The world needs you to.

So to reiterate my point from earlier, do your homework. Question whatever you come across and bring a healthy level of skepticism to your education. As far as the industry is concerned, if something is being marketed to you and is targeting your self-esteem and promising its product will be the solution to your personal happiness or worth, then ignore it. Chances are it is creating a codependency between your self-worth and its product or service. It or they want you to buy their product and feel good about it so that you'll tell your friends and they'll buy their products as well.

This isn't to say that sometimes products or services can give you the helping hand you may need to establish a healthy relationship with yourself, food, exercise, or maybe with others. That's fine; I know a bucketload of either books, courses, or coaches that have really helped me see things that I otherwise would never have seen and then provided necessary steps of action and discovery to go about making a change. These types of guides or teachers are necessary and healthy. The largest concern comes not with dependency but the codependency that either people or products can knowingly or unknowingly create.

One of the best things you can do for long-term health when it comes to the fitness industry is make the distinction between what products and services are being marketed to you for the benefit of the seller (win:lose), which ones are there to help you (win:win) and which ones are for the long-term health, happiness, and education of everyone involved (win:win:win).

The reason why the win:win:win options are the best is because they are not just a win for the person providing the service and the person receiving it but also a win for those involved in their home life, their work life, and if it is based in education it will also make an impact on their kids and the next generation.

When we educate rather than just demonstrate health, we make real long-term change because it becomes intergenerational.

In short, look for win:win:wins. Your kids will thank you.

The Human Interaction Model

A couple of years ago, a model called Codependent Patterns was introduced. Later on when teaching it, I had a client exclaim she had also been taught this model by a therapist who called it the Human Interaction Model. Let's be clear; I am no therapist, and this isn't my model. What this model clearly shows us is how easy it is to create relationships with people or things that keep us unfulfilled, hopeless, and living in fear.

The Human Interaction Model has four different levels:

1. Codependent
2. Dependent
3. Independent
4. Interdependent

For the sake of the exercise, we are going to keep their numbers but flip their order so that they look like this:

4. Interdependent
3. Independent
2. Dependent
1. Codependent

INTERDEPENDENT - ADAPTIVE

INDEPENDENT - CREATIVE

DEPENDENT

↑ FEEDBACK ↑   • LOVE
• EDUCATION

CO-DEPENDENT

• PRISONER   RESCUER   • FEAR
• BLAME   • LIMITING
                                     BELIEFS

DRAMA
CYCLE

VICTIM   AGGRESSOR

There are a multitude of reasons as to why somebody would gravitate to a particular level. A couple of examples would be childhood patterns and conditioning, conditional self-worth, and the ways in which we communicate love. We also have different levels for different areas of our lives. For example, someone could be interdependent when it comes to business but codependent when it comes to their health. Once again, this is a fluid and dynamic model like all the models I share with you in this book. We use it as a guide to see where we are and where we want to be and then plan how to get there.

The levels are not inherently bad or necessarily unhealthy. They are just pointing to how we interact with other people and things out there in the world.

Codependency

In a codependent relationship there will be three things or kinds of people. A victim, an aggressor, and a rescuer. The reason why this is a codependent stage is because each person or thing is depending on the other two to uphold its identity. A victim needs an aggressor, a rescuer needs a victim, an aggressor needs a rescuer and vice versa. This is called the Drama Cycle.

This can be used in many different ways with many different examples, one of which could be an intimate relationship and another could be a relationship at work.

My examples are going to revolve around the fitness industry and also our relationship with things.

People stay in this relationship out of fear and limiting beliefs. Here is a simple example from the fitness industry.

Somebody wants to lose weight, and so they go to a new trainer and ask them to help them lose 20 kg.

They complain about always being overweight and always struggling with losing it. They say they are sick of it and really want someone to motivate them to lose the weight.

Insert motivating trainer who prides themselves on helping people lose weight. The trainer runs this person through a 12-week program, and they lose 9 kg in 12 weeks.

Not quite 20, but for the first time, the overweight person has seen a drastic change. They associate their results with the motivating trainer who pushed them through the workout, told them what to eat, and called them up when they didn't come in.

Let's pause here—what can we see? I can see someone who is potentially a victim to their weight (the aggressor) and the trainer is there to rescue them from the aggressor. The trainer isn't aware that they find so much value and personal worth out of helping people, and so they really pride themselves on helping people achieve their goal because it feeds a condition they have put on their self-esteem.

The trainer is overly responsible and goes above and beyond and will do anything to get results for their client. Which, they did get. On face value, all appears good in the world. The client tells all their friends about how caring and supportive their trainer is and gives an awesome testimonial so that the trainer can help more people.

The client is being rescued from their aggressor, which is their weight. One of the mental challenges for someone at this stage is that if they aren't able to move upward to the next level of "dependent" then they are going to struggle to lose the rest of the weight. Somewhere in their unconscious they have identified as a victim, so they need the aggressor to help them uphold that identity.

Curve ball—you could have a client who when they were younger, were told by their father that women like that don't go after men like us. Men like what? Overweight men, son. We are just invisible to them. Or "Men are liars, and your father left me for a younger skinnier bitch who hates us."

If for some reason, these types of things were said, remembered, and then created into a belief by the client at a younger age, then there are so many possibilities as to why someone may struggle to lose weight or find self-worth. As a trainer, you are to support and guide your client to the best of your abilities. This is also why I say the trainer is not responsible for the client's results. There is so much going on that the trainer may not be able to see. It is also not the trainer's job to go into therapy, and this is why I say not everyone is ready to get their result because not everyone is aware of what is creating an identity that they don't know about.

So, sure, it is challenging, and it can be complex. This is why we need to clear the crap in the way that is stopping us from living the life that we want to live.

Okay, let's resume—so say the client who has lost the weight is still training with the trainer six months later. They have lost a further 5 kg but not much else is budging. Not like in the first 12 weeks. The client may start looking for a new rescuer or maybe bring back the old aggressor. They haven't broken away from the old identity, and they feel like a 15 kg lighter fraud.

Eventually the client slows down the number of times they train until they have some small distraction happen in life, which gives them the out they need to go back to how things were. To go back to some of the order before the chaos.

When people commit to changing their life by doing something like losing weight, they are committing to leaving their old world behind. They are committed to learning new behaviors, new beliefs, new thoughts, new friends, and sometimes a new spouse. For a lot of people, that is a lot to give up. Until they realize that they are giving up their best life for the one they have settled for.

Everything is a trade-off.

So how do we move from codependent to dependent? In this circumstance the trainer supports that transition for the client through education and love. Once again that can look different for each person, and it is important to remember that this is a process; there is no finish line. The education is a continual learning and developing on top of the learning, and the love part involves patience, listening, lack of judgment, and support.

We all have the capacity to be codependent in at least one area of our life. In order to ask for help, we are asking to be rescued. We have a problem (the aggressor), and we are victims to it. The key difference here is whether we want to evolve and free ourselves from the old identity and also whether the person who is helping us has the ability and ego strength to help us develop. A good coach will get you to a point where you no longer need them, whether a fitness coach, a relationship coach, or a business coach. You may still interact and learn from them, you just no longer lean on them in the way you did when you started out.

Developing independence or interdependence in one area doesn't necessarily cross over to others. Where a businessperson is independent or interdependent with marketing and sales, they may be in a codependent relationship with their accountant when it comes to taxation. They also may never want to develop past that stage and be more than happy to keep the relationship codependent.

It is when we unwillingly stay in a codependent relationship in order to keep an identity that may be harmful in the long term that it becomes an issue. It is also not empowering for a trainer to keep a client in this space. It is very much the opposite; the trainer is disempowering them. They are taking away their personal power and building conditions on their achievements.

As I have explained, people can be in a codependent relationship with other people, but they can also be in a codependent relationship with objects or other things out there in the world.

"I can't start my day without my coffee."

I (the victim) am not able to deal with the unknowns of the day (the aggressor) without my morning coffee (the rescuer).

People do it with coffee, they do it with knee sleeves, or training equipment, and they can do it with alcohol. I can think of a few people who need a few drinks in order to dance or talk to the girl across the bar.

Dependency

As we develop and move up the model, we move into dependency. On face of it, dependency can seem like a bad thing; however, it is extremely natural. People may like to brag that they have never had to depend on anyone; however, I am sure they didn't go and pump their own petrol/gas from another country and then bring it back to their country to put it in the car that they built.

When I turn the light on, I depend on the electricity company to do their job. Dependency is the first step after the drama cycle. We still lean on people and things; however, we are not powerless without them. In the above example of the client losing weight, the trainer would continually and lovingly prod the client in the right direction, giving them opportunities to step up and take responsibility. They would still show them and teach them what to eat, instruct them through exercises, and check in from time to time, but most importantly, they will give the client an opportunity to really step up and start owning their decisions and ultimately start taking responsibility for their health.

The subtle opportunities to offer personal ownership can almost fly under the radar. When you hear a client say something like "you made me do burpees," it may seem harmless, but that person is communicating that they are only doing it because you made them. It almost sounds like a parent-child relationship.

"You made me go to my room."

I have never made anyone do burpees. I have programmed them, I have encouraged them, but at no point have I ever grabbed someone by the collar or held their family at gunpoint until they flopped onto the floor into a sweaty mess for five reps.

Don't blame me for your results.

As individuals we have multiple opportunities every day to own our shit, to really start to see when we are not being responsible for our language and our actions. You did the burpees, you got your ass up out of bed, and you ate the chocolate. No one made you do anything. When I make you do something and you oblige, I strip you of your power to choose. When I do that, I own you. All this insecure behavior is left behind in the codependent space. In dependency, you are making your first steps to clearing the crap and owning your shit.

Independency

At the independent level, we still depend on others; the difference is that we are able to depend on ourselves first. This is why it is called INdependent. We go inward for dependency and then outward. We lean on our own decision-making process, our self-esteem, and the strength of others. We want someone around for the sake of having someone around. We don't need somebody else's approval to feel good about ourselves and are cautious of people who come across like they are still intertwined in the drama cycle. For the most part, at this level people operate at a healthy level of responsibility.

Once again, all this is dependent upon the healthiness of the individual, which changes from day to day and week to week. This is fluid and dynamic. Even at this level, under a lot of stress you may find yourself regressing back to codependent behaviors.

One of the key characteristics for people at this stage is that they are often creative when it comes to their thinking and problem solving. To use a quick example from before, if the lights aren't working due to a power outage at night, they have a backup generator ready to go, a torch, and some candles on hand. An easy way to make a distinction is that a 12-year-old child may not be thinking about any of this (for many reasons) and thus will be dependent or codependent on their parents to bring forward a solution to the situation.

In a training scenario, a client may still take recommendations, plans, and advice from their coach; they are just able to own their health and be creative with the decisions they make with relation to the problems and situations that arise. If they are away on holidays, they choose to stay active and are able to find ways to do that which may also include going to the gym. A codependent person will say they couldn't go to the gym because their trainer wasn't there whereas a dependent person may join a class as they want to exercise but may not feel fully competent on knowing what to program or back themselves to keep the intensity. Independent and interdependent individuals may also attend classes if they choose to. The key difference is that they are choosing to; it isn't the only option available for them.

We level up to independent when we lean into self-love, trust in self, and confidence in building confidence. The interesting thing about trust is that people here trust themselves to be able to either complete the pursued goal or be able to deal with the fall out that comes from failing. Often at the lower levels, it isn't that they don't trust themselves to achieve a set goal; it is that they don't trust themselves to be able to deal with failing the goal and the unknown that comes with that.

Interdependency

At the interdependent level of relationship, individuals are completely adaptive, regardless of the environment, the circumstance, and challenges they are able to adapt and overcome. They don't believe in a lack of resources but rather that people are unresourceful.

An example of the thinking associated with this level can be seen in relationships. At a lower level, you may see or hear things such as "You complete me." At the interdependent level, that becomes "I am complete, and I choose you."

There is no dependency on another but rather a choice to be there with them, not for them. This same sentiment can extend to a coach–client relationship, a work relationship, and so on. What this is really saying is out of being anywhere and doing anything in the world, I am choosing to show up here today, with you, now.

Imagine people choosing to be with you out of a desire to be with you rather than needing you to feel complete. We can take this same energy to our training, to our health, to our family relations. With another love and education we can take it to everything.

The lower stages are "I am not enough, so I need you." The higher stages are "I am enough, and I choose you."

The "you" in those sentences can be a relationship, a nutrition plan, a goal, or a career. If you think about it, a lot of careers are chosen based on wanting to keep people's parents happy. And for some people, if they were to leave that career they would disappoint their parents. They are keeping the job because they have associated love with making their caretakers happy, not making themselves happy. It is a codependency based on the idea that I am not enough without their approval, and their approval is based on me having or succeeding at this job.

Interdependence is living life by choice and by personal design. It is being able to adapt to a situation and not see good or bad but rather a wider perspective on each situation and have a deeper long-term purpose. They live life by intention rather than for attention. To live life by intention is to make decisions based off what you have decided is a worthy purpose to live your life for. To live by attention is to allow attention to govern your decisions. This can be in the form of wanting attention or making decisions to avoid attention. Both are governed by attention, not intention.

At the interdependence stage, people see success and failure as a process rather than a black-and-white, good-or-bad situation. For example, someone who gets injured will use it as an opportunity to learn more about their body, the injury, how to prevent it, where their weaknesses are that may have caused the injury, and how they are able to learn from the injury. How many sport stars have come back from injuries bigger, faster, and stronger? How many sport stars have had career-ending injuries and gone on to become a positive influence in other areas such as public speaking or for a bigger cause than sport, like being conservationists and then use their influence to make a bigger impact?

People at lower stages see the injury as bad and can potentially become a victim to it. Having a good or bad perspective on something is a static way to view an event. Developing a dynamic and process perspective allows us to see that things that may initially appear bad make way for opportunity for good and vice versa.

There is a story about a Chinese farmer that helps illustrate this point.

A farmer purchases a horse and a couple of weeks later the horse runs away. His neighbor comes over and says, "How unlucky is that?"

The farmer replies, "Who am I to know about luck?"

Two days later the horse comes back with three other horses.

"How lucky is that?" says the neighbor. "First it ran away and then it came back with three other horses."

The farmer replies, "Who am I to know about luck?"

 The next day the farmer's son is riding one of the new horses, and he gets thrown off it and breaks his leg.

"How unlucky is that? Now he can't help you on the farm," says the neighbor.

"Who am I to know about luck?"

A week later the emperor's men go to all the farms and take every able-bodied young man to fight in a war. The farmer's son, however, cannot walk.

How lucky is that?

The fitness industry can be guilty of marketing to people's insecurities and building co-dependencies to create repeat customers who simply must have their products or services; otherwise, they would be devoid of self-worth and confidence.

Your job is to take your power back, away from those who simply do not care about you and begin to make decisions based off your long-term happiness and education. In doing so you not only improve your own Health IQ, but you consequently challenge everyone around you to step up as well. Playing small serves no one. Playing victim only serves those who want to keep you there. Taking personal responsibility is how we change the world, one person at a time and never afraid of the long game. The industry is selling quick fixes to complex problems. They are selling physical solutions to mental and emotional struggles. Physical solutions become a by-product of working on all of you, mind and body.

Ego says, "When everything falls into place, I will be at peace."

Spirit says, "When I am at peace, everything will fall into place."

The Life Athlete

My personal challenge to you is to become what I call a "life athlete."

A life athlete is somebody who looks at what they want to achieve in life and then goes about training their mind and training their body to allow them to do that. Life athletes don't just hit and celebrate personal records (PRs) in the gym; life athletes pursue life PRs.

A life athlete is once again different for each individual. Some life athletes are professional body builders. Others can be hobby hikers or gardeners. My dad is a life athlete. He has a goal to play field hockey for Australia. He knows there is an over-75 age group. So he figures if he keeps playing, by then people will either have retired or they will have kicked the bucket. So at the time of this writing, he is 62 and still runs around on a field twice a week. He is able to play with his grandchildren and do all the basic physical tasks that are required of him to live the life he wants.

Being a life athlete isn't about what you look like. As we have already established, the fitness industry is simply dressed up as the beauty industry, and it has lead a large majority of people to believe that happiness is on the other side of an image. In my experience that is only fleeting, and one could argue that it isn't true happiness. Like just about anything taken to an extreme, pursuing an image can become an extreme addiction, but because it is in the "health industry," we may not perceive it as being as bad as a drug, gambling, or food addiction.

What you look like is a by-product of what you do, think, and eat. When we are a life athlete, we train for performance and the ability to live our best life outside of the gym. We have a belief that your one hour in the gym must positively impact your 23 hours outside of the gym; otherwise, it is a cost. It is no longer an investment. If what we do in the gym isn't allowing us to become better fathers, mothers, accountants, builders, uncles, hobby hikers, adventurers, or whatever is linked to our life goals, then what is the point?

The key idea here is to use the gym and fitness industry; don't let the gym and fitness industry use and abuse you. Life athletes develop all of themselves, not just their body. They see everyone who comes into their environment as someone on a journey and sees them as they are. There is no judgment or silent egotistical competition. They understand that everyone is simply unfolding at their own rate. They understand that they also didn't know what a deadlift or a barbell or a rower was at some point.

Life athletes see the bigger picture and use the gym and exercise to allow them to live it.

If we don't have our training regime in correlation to our life goals, then too often it is easy to fall into the category of out exercising our goals. When the goal is to generally get fitter or stronger, then we start to risk exercising for exercising's sake. Of course this is perceived to be better than sitting on a couch and never doing anything, and maybe it is a part of where someone needs to start in order to become a life athlete, but at some point, the individual will grow tired of just smashing themselves in the gym for the sake of it, burning calories because they were told that's what was important. It's not. It's a by-product of keeping healthy for a purpose-driven life.

If we aren't careful, people just chase the sweats. They chase the point of not being able to breathe and settle for a workout that was really hard. Every time. This is not performance. This is borderline machoism. High-level athletes do not train like this. Their programming is tapered and designed to be able to perform without injury. For the most part, the general population is going to the gym with this idea of needing to smash it three to six days a week without good recovery practices in place, no periodization, and no direct training goal.

When the rule of thumb is go hard or go home, sometimes it is good to go home. So that the next day, when you come in, you can go hard. Training isn't always exercise.

This brings forward the importance of goals. I am not talking about the general goals that we circle on a pretraining questionnaire. I am talking about purposeful, worthy goals that give meaning to the reason why we train, which aren't based on conditions and other people's approval.

Goals can compel us to want to go to the gym or go for a run or go to yoga because we see that it is the vehicle that takes us away from where we don't want to be and takes us to where we want to go. I have heard over the years that exercise has helped people keep anxiety or depression at arm's length. Although there are multiple studies that show the positive effects that exercise has on these conditions among many others, if we aren't careful, they will not keep them at bay. They either prolong them from getting worse or they distract us from dealing with what we may need to face in order to overcome and move through them.

Exercise alone isn't the answer. It is a factor in the solution of a multifaceted problem. If we lean on exercise too much then, like on drugs or alcohol, it can become the go-to coping mechanism when we feel anxiety or depression coming on. In the short term, this sounds like a great idea. Over the long term, it can become an unhealthy coping mechanism. We start off small by going for a run or to the gym, and we see some positive change in our mental state and body. Then over time we have the same things that trigger us to feel that initial feeling either in the outside world or in our thoughts about the outside world, so we go to the gym again. Soon enough we find ourselves going to the gym multiple times a day to deal with the "demons" until one day we either burn out or injure ourselves. Then when this happens, we have to now face our demons because our coping mechanism has been taking away from us not realizing that it was us that took it away by abusing something that was part of the solution and not the solution.

Exercise is so beneficial for mental health. It's just that by itself it isn't the long-term antidote to an internal problem. This isn't a book about overcoming anxiety, and I am not a therapist. The things I don't point at in this book will no doubt have an effect on some poor mental health, but my suggestion is to not stop here, continue learning as much about yourself as possible.

In order to be life athletes, we must have goals and targets in our life that we want to work toward and achieve. Sometimes we can fall into the idea that any goal is better than no goal. This can be argued both ways. One thing to consider is that if you don't know what you want and you just start working toward an arbitrary goal, then chances are it is someone else's goal, and while you are focused on achieving that, you aren't able to give yourself space to go deep inside and decide what truly is important to you. Most people's goals are distractions from their purpose, and most people's salaries are hush money for their dreams.

So to become a life athlete who smashes life PRs, we have to set some targets and goals that mean something to us. Unlike some old-school style of thinking, we don't achieve something then become it. We achieve by becoming it, and we become it by daily action toward being an individual who lives their life in congruence with what's most important to them. This is the difference between living with intention rather than living for attention.

When we live with intention, we enable our decisions to be governed by an overarching purpose that has deep meaning to us. It allows us to make distinctions about long-term happiness over short-term happiness. Decisions governed by intention don't choose short-term pleasure for long-term pain; they see value in playing the long game no matter what their purpose is and instead choose short-term pain for long-term pleasure. When we are living in congruence with a deeper meaning, we don't have to be motivated or inspired, and we don't just take action when we feel like it. We have a deeper intrinsic drive that allows us to see the big picture and deploy patience to something worth obtaining.

The opposite, which is to live for attention, can be those who constantly seek the attention or approval of others, but it can also be those who hide from the attention. Both are making decisions governed by attention. Avoiding attention or seeking it is the same thing. The former can be obvious and also very subtle, the latter isn't obvious at all.

With the former, people will try to set goals and show their achievements in hope of some form of external validation, even though they will deny that they do that often say they do it for themselves and some people may. It is when we are able to step back and look at our goals and our behaviors that we start to see a pattern that links to the approval of others, whether they be individuals or a particular group of people. This can often be shamed or frowned upon, when in reality, most people haven't been taught how to find that approval within. They weren't taught that what they think of themselves is more important than what others think of them. They may not trust themselves, so they seek the approval of others to know that they are on the right track and therefore safe. It is neither good nor bad; the issue arises when it blindly influences our goal because we will get to the end and still feel unfulfilled.

In the latter case, people will often make decisions to avoid the limelight and avoid the attention of others. If these decisions are being governed by attention, then they are still stemming from attention. It is the same thing as doing things for attention. These people may avoid making decisions that are important to them to avoid attention or may even perform at a lower level just to fly under the radar. Attention, not intention, is still the governing principle in their decisions. They may have associated attention with being in trouble or they may discount themselves and have low self-confidence, and so they wish to not be seen because for them, not being seen means they are safe.

One key difference between living in intention and living for attention is where we get permission. People who live in congruence with their intentions seek permission from within. They don't need somebody else to give them permission to pursue what is important to them. They have a healthy sense of internal authority and see that what they want is already there and go about it patiently (and sometimes impatiently). Those who live for attention, however, will continue to seek permission externally. They are the ones who are waiting to be saved by someone; they are the ones who will ask other people for permission before pursuing something. There is a subtle sense of lack of responsibility in those who are living for attention as they seek to get permission from someone, as if the other person somehow knows what is best for them. In some cases, this may be true. When it comes to surgeons, that would make sense. When it comes to life decisions about what we want, then that's when we can catch ourselves giving away our power and living for the attention of others or the avoidance of the attention of others. Sometimes, attention is simply dressed up as approval.

When we are able to observe these governing influences in our behavior, we have the opportunity to step back and truly ask what is important to us. Ask the questions, am I being true to what is important to me? What is it that I really fear? Are my goals aligned with my values or are they aligned with the approval of others? When we make decisions based off what other people think or may think, then we fall into some murky waters. We are not in control of what others may think about us.

There is a passage I came across that was shared on social media that said,

"I read a book that blew my mind. The main character goes crazy when he realizes that no one really knows him."

The gist is that the person you think of as "yourself" exists only for you. And even *you* don't really know who that is. Every person you meet, have a relationship with, or make eye contact in the street with, creates a different version of "you" in their heads. You're not the same person to your mom, your dad, and your siblings that you are to your coworkers, your neighbors, or your friends. There are a thousand different versions of yourself out there, in people's minds. A "you" exists in each version, and yet your "you," "yourself," isn't really "someone" at all.

This feeds directly to the quote from Thomas Cooley: "I am not who you think I am; I am not who I think I am; I am who I think you think I am."

When we make decisions governed by attention, we are giving weight to other people's potential opinion of us, on what may be best for us or what our personal worth is in the eyes of someone else. We may neglect to realize that all their opinions (like ours) are often heavily filtered by who they think we are and their own biases that they may not even see. Then, if we aren't aware, we live by their rules, constantly being pulled here and there in order to seek externally what is already within us.

One more story that describes this point so well was told by Wayne Dyer.

A man was out in the front of his house looking for his watch. His neighbor noticed him searching in the garden and asked him what he was doing. "I am looking for my watch," he told his neighbor. The neighbor offered to help him look for it as it was getting late, and the sun was not too far from setting. After an hour or so of looking for this watch and with little sunlight left, the neighbor turned and asked the watch owner where he'd last had his watch. "I last had it inside the house," said the watch's owner.

"Well, if you lost it inside, why are you looking outside for it?"

Too often we go looking outside for things we lost inside. Yet another difference between living in intention and living for attention.

Often it is by digging into our goals that we are able to uncover the truth. On the face of it we can trick ourselves into the "nice guy/girl" paradigm. In this paradigm, people have tricked themselves into thinking that everything they do is pure and from a good place, and they could never do anything wrong and if they did it wouldn't be there fault. They are stuck in the idea that if the other person was to think bad of them then they would be a bad person, so they trick themselves into always being the good guy/girl not realizing that this is simply from a place of attention. The attention of others and the weight of their opinion. I will go through this a bit deeper in the mind part of the book.

To conclude, the life athlete has a deeper drive that comes through them and leads them to make decisions from a place of intention rather than for attention. Intention is the deep power that allows them to direct their energy to a particular source and see it through to the end or wherever necessary because it isn't dependent upon outside approval or permission.

Life athletes set and pursue life PRs because they live life on their terms. People often mistake this as just a heap of selfish people going around only caring about themselves and putting everyone else last and themselves first. Firstly, selfishness is a precursor to selflessness. Secondly, when we look after ourselves, we no longer put the burden of our well-being in the hands of someone else. We build a healthy level of responsibility for our health and our life and in turn encourage others to do the same. True helping is living the life and being the example. That wouldn't be the reason to live life on your terms; it is a by-product. When people see you take ownership of your health and your life, it inspires them to do the same thing. Some people will rebel against it, let them. A healthy life athlete can live their life along with other people who are on different journeys. They understand every person is developing and unfolding at their own rate. This is called being in a choice-based relationship, whether it is an intimate relationship, a platonic relationship, or a working relationship. In a choice-based relationship, you have made the decision that what the other person does and where the other person is in their life is just where they are. Since you don't have to conform to their values and beliefs, you recognize that they don't have to conform to yours. And if they do, it could likely mean you are projecting what is important to you onto them. This is a sign of a need-based relationship. In short, a need-based relationship is where someone needs to behave or act in a particular way in order to get your love and approval. You need them to do particular things and live by a particular set of values in order for you to love them or accept them in your life. What is interesting about this is that it is often a projection of our own values and beliefs that they have to behave like in order for us to love them. If they behave like us, then we will love them, which is truly only loving ourselves. Being in a choice-based relationship may mean we spend less time with someone; we respect where they are at and what they are doing; we are simply just working on what is most important to us and allowing them to do the same.

This may mean that some people will stop being your friends, let them. Some people will say nasty things about you, let them. Some people may even go to great lengths in an attempt to make you feel the pain they feel, let them. It is all a reflection and projection of where they are at, not you. We hate what we don't understand. The other key point here to remember that difficult people are just hurt people and hurt people, hurt people. They are living life by their map and their rules and by you doing what you are doing, you are defying the rules and conditions of their map of reality. This doesn't mean you are doing anything wrong at all. It means they aren't taking responsibility for what's in their control and what they have power over. Life athletes live life by their map, not other people's. Live life on your terms and let everyone else do the same.

The last thing I want to say with regard to becoming a life athlete is that there is nothing wrong with being a beginner. There is no shame in not knowing, there is no shame in starting out later in life, and there is no shame in any stage of learning. Just start, where you are, with what you have. We all have to be a beginner at some point if we want to get good at it.

Health IQ

After leaving my first job in a gym that I had worked at for over six years, I went about addressing coaching and fitness from a different angle. For years I had told people what to do, told them what to eat, and even called them up when they didn't show up and motivated them to come back in and keep training. I was really good at it; I knew my stuff and people got results.

Then, slowly, after a while they would revert back to where they started. Something would happen; they would move house or get an injury or change jobs, and they would go back to the same habits as before. Then, the cycle would continue; they would come in, I would train them, tell them what to eat and we would get results again. After doing this for several years, I grew tired of it. Hardly anybody was achieving their results and then neither keeping them nor surpassing them. Hardly anyone was progressing. What I later learned was how codependent the relationship I had with the clients was, but more importantly, I wasn't educating them. They would simply revert back to old behaviors and habits.

When I left the first job, I decided I wanted to start an educational company, not an exercise company. The difference that made the difference is when I realized that I am not in the health industry teaching people; I am in the people industry teaching health, teaching people to develop what I call their Health IQ. At first, the concept of Health IQ was not much but a nice sentiment. Although I roughly knew what I was referring to and what it meant, it wasn't until I was later challenged by a mentor to break down what Health IQ was, how it could be measured, and how people can develop it that I was able to put together a map that allows people to do just that.

What Is Health IQ?

Health IQ (HIQ from here on) is measured in three different areas; mind-set, movement, and nutrition. HIQ is a measurement of how well we know our body, mind, and soul. And it goes past just fitness and our ability to follow a diet plan and includes living in alignment with our personal values and integrity. It is understanding how food, movement, and our thoughts impact our health and overall life. This is going to be different for each person because we have different goals and value different experiences. HIQ is quite unique to the individual because how nutrition affects your body will differ from the next person. You will have different goals and also enjoy different life experiences.

Although we are all human and have so many similarities, we still have so many differences that need to be reflected in how well we know ourselves.

On the HIQ Map, each area has three levels or stages. There is a fourth stage that isn't shown on the map which is the pre-stage to the HIQ Map. Otherwise known as "asleep." In pre-stage, people aren't aware that they need to develop their mental health, nutrition, or physical body. They are often in a static stage of living and are content with things just plodding along as they are until something occurs where they absolutely have to make a change. They are walking around asleep until something or someone wakes them up out of it.

The first stage of each is the awareness stage. It is where people are aware they want to or feel they need to develop that stage, and it can often be the hardest stage to work through. At this stage across the three areas, we are starting out as a beginner in many ways. One of the important things to remember is that there is nothing wrong with being a beginner. In fact being a beginner at something is a necessity to being a master at something. Being 50 years old isn't too late to learn about nutrition, and 19 isn't too young to learn about mind-set. There is no age by which you should have known all or any of this. The beginner stage simply means that you are beginning. It's where we become increasingly competent at whatever we are working at even though it takes a lot of work.

The stage that best suits you is governed by your overarching goal. We will cover this in a later chapter as we want to set a compelling target to aim toward; what is important to grasp now is that the highest stage isn't always the best stage for everyone. The map isn't set up in a way to say that the top stage is any better than the first stage. All stages serve a purpose and will be relevant for different people at different stages. For example, the attention and trade-offs that are required of you to get to the highest stage of physical mastery, nutritional accuracy, and mindful abundance may be taking away from your goal of writing a book, starting a family, or growing a business. The HIQ Map allows us to see the flexibility and stages required to be able to smash our life PRs and live our life on our terms. Not just be fit and lean for Instagram. It's a hard trade-off, I know.

The HIQ Map

The HIQ Map was designed in a specific way to show people a path of development as well as a step-by-step process on how to get there. The map is a tool and a resource for your goals rather than a goal itself. The whole idea behind a life athlete is to set goals in life and crush them. This map supports the stages of where you need to be to be able to do just that. When we shift our focus to the map and conquering the map becomes the goal, then we have lost the point of the map.

Each stage is flexible and has a range. We will all have a bandwidth that we operate in which shows our baseline or average, our peak state, and also our stress anchor. This reflects how we operate under stress and the habits we may drop down to in times of stress as well as peak states we reach when we feel secure and safe.

As mentioned before, the three areas of the map are mind-set, movement, and nutrition. Another way to think of these three are mind, move, mouth.

Each of these areas of health has three stages. Those stages are as follows:

Mind-set—student, scholar, sage
Movement—safe, strong, sexy
Mouth—simple, sustainable, specific

Although I will break down these areas more in their corresponding chapters, a good way to think of the three stages is to understand the conscious competence scale.

The Conscious Competence Scale

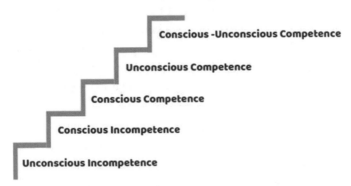

Conscious -Unconscious Competence

Unconscious Competence

Conscious Competence

Conscious Incompetence

Unconscious Incompetence

There are five levels to the conscious competence scale. I have given the everyday example of driving as well as where these levels fit into the HIQ Map.

The first level is unconscious incompetence. At this level, people aren't aware of what they aren't good at. An easy example of this is driving. When we are young, we aren't aware just how challenging driving is and how bad we are at it, until we do it ourselves. This is also the pre-stage or the sleeping stage of the HIQ Map. People here have a poor HIQ level but are unaware of it.

The second level is conscious incompetence. At this level we realize how bad we are at said task. In the driving example, this is where we would spend the majority of our time learning to gain competency. We have to focus hard on all the details we are learning; however, we are in a stage of being conscious of our incompetence. These are the beginning stages of the HIQ Map. Here we have to focus really hard at being competent at our thoughts (mind), the way we move and our body's intelligence (move), and make conscious decisions with food (mouth).

The third level is conscious competence. At this level we are able to carry out the task competently but are heavily focused on the task at hand and require there to be minimal to no distractions. This would be the early stage of our driving life where we are able to go out on the road by ourselves; however, we have to maintain focus of the task. For the HIQ Map, this is where we start to really build consistency with our thoughts and beliefs and have them work for us and not against us (mind), it is where we build a strong relationship with our body and its profound ability (move), and where our healthy nutritional decisions start to feel natural. We can spend up to a number of years at this stage so that we can move on to the following stage. The 10,000-hour rule comes online mostly during this stage. There is a big difference between 10,000 hours of practice and 10,000 hours of conscious practice.

The fourth level is unconscious competence. At this level people are able to carry out said tasks with ease and finesse. Often people at this level at their respective skill can make what seems to be impossible, possible. And they often make it look easy. For drivers, this means they are able to scan the horizon for potential dangers, remember which directions they need to take, talk to the passengers, and listen out for any dangers, and not be aware that they are doing any and all of these things all at once. For the HIQ Map, it means complete mind emptiness and nonattachment (mind), physical mastery, and freedom of movement (move), and nutritional flexibility and knowledge (mouth). To be at this stage, the person would have spent thousands of hours of conscious practice of their craft to be able to do what they do so effortlessly.

The fifth and relatively unknown level is conscious unconscious competence. This is the teacher level—someone who has brought consciousness to what they do unconsciously so that they are able to break it down and teach their competence to someone else. It is the driver understanding how they do all those things at once and being able to break it down into consumable information chunks for the person they are teaching. For the HIQ Map, it means understanding the importance of all stages and being able to breakdown step by step how they developed to where they are at in order to help other people do the same. This is why those who have climbed to the highest position in their field be it Brazilian jiujitsu or business will talk about the long game and being patient by taking things step by step.

All these levels can be seen within the HIQ model and the nutrition grading.

Each level, including the unconscious incompetence level, is as important as the other. As you develop through the levels, you transcend and include the level you just moved through. What this means is that you aren't able to skip ahead without doing the work. You aren't able to become consciously competent at something if you aren't aware of it and then aware of how bad you are at it and then consciously work at it to become competent at it. This the same rule for mastering the piano as it is for becoming a world-class surgeon.

Let's take a closer look at the conscious competence scale and how it integrates with the HIQ Map with regard to nutrition (mouth).

When somebody first becomes aware of the importance and power that food has they start to move from the sleeping unconscious incompetence stage to the very early conscious incompetence stage. This is where people who first move into the "simple" stage of the HIQ are starting out. By taking one step at a time and in small chunks, over time, that person can become consciously competent through education and patience. Often, a lack of patience is what causes people to yo-yo. They are improving, just not at the rate they are "supposed to." This then can cause the person to give up because they think they are failing. Only to regather themselves in a few months or years to try again. Unfortunately, they often try again with the same attitude that caused them to stop the first time. But with support, guidance, and persistence the individual can develop their skills and move on to the next level.

This is one of the reasons why I am more interested in receiving a letter in three years about how clients have changed their lives and the experiences some of them have had compared to the before-and-after "transformation" in 12 weeks. The three-year letter promotes patience and supports the values associated with long-term vision.

Once the person has moved into conscious competence, they begin to become more consistent with their work and what used to be a lot of effort is starting to become habitual. They build a sustainable approach to nutrition through education and execution of plans. This will usually include some trial and error, which will initially look like failure, but overtime will be seen as research. This is the "sustainable" stage in the HIQ model.

Over years of spending time at this stage, learning and trying new things and gaining experience, the individual can move into the unconscious competence stage where they have wired their behaviors and thoughts after hours and hours and years and years of conscious repetition. They have gained flexibility with nutrition and have the ability to be extremely precise with their portions and meals and yet still keep the ability to dial back and relax more without feeling guilty. They have power of food rather than food having power over them.

In order for someone to reach the level of conscious unconscious competence, they must now integrate the mind and body together with belief structures, patience, and a healthy level of responsibility to really be able to teach people how to develop themselves. For most people, this level just simply isn't necessary when it comes to teaching nutrition precision. Hence why it is important to operate at a level that suits your life goals.

In the nutrition chapter, you will learn about the nutrition-grading model and see how the conscious competence model has been integrated into both the HIQ model and the nutrition grading model.

I decided to call it the HIQ Map and not a model because it should help you map where you need to be and what you need to do in order to achieve what you want. It helps to show where we may be weak within any of the three areas and how to get to a higher level that will better support your life goals.

Because there is a vast range of life goals and it would be nearly (if not) impossible to fit them all into a model, it will take some work at your end to figure out just where you need to be to best suit your intended target. This means that as you continue on your path to achieving what's most important to you, continually check back in to see if your habits, behaviors, and thoughts are in congruence with where you have suggested you need to be on the map.

The map simply points out the stages and what is required of people to move to that stage. It is up to you to make the decision as to where you are and where you need to be to reach your intended target. Make no mistake that all three areas are integral to success in any area of health that we want to develop. To neglect one is to neglect our potential. Often people will have one area of strength, one area of competence, and one area they neglect. When we are able to bring harmony and consistency to all three of these areas, we are able to pursue just about anything in life that is humanly possible.

As with everything in life, there are always trade-offs. When we start to invest time in one area of our development, that time doesn't just come out of nowhere. We have to get it from somewhere. Sometimes the trade-off is less trash TV. Sometimes the trade-off is quitting your job. Other times the trade-off is family time or even our mental health. We choose the trade-off. So if you have set a target of achieving the highest level in all three areas, just be aware of what you are inadvertently choosing. Time just doesn't come out of nowhere and you can't make more of it.

For someone who is at a stage in their life and just wants to be able to do whatever they want, whenever the opportunity comes up, then being consistent in the midrange on all three areas of health is best. An example of such a person is someone who enjoys being able to jump into social or semi-competitive sports or maybe an obstacle course race without having to do a complete makeover of their life. They would simply tailor their training for somewhere between 10 to 15 weeks to be able to get the most out of a desired event or competition. They enjoy the flexibility of being able to experience different ways to test their mind and body without having to go all in on one thing for years and years. Often this person is seen as a jack-of-all-trades and in the past has even been frowned upon.

In more recent years, functional training has given this type of life athlete a reprieve as they enjoy the fruits from a magnitude of different endeavors and are okay with never reaching the peak of any particular sport or competition. They build mastery over choice and flexibility rather than mastery over a sport.

If we had a population who all averaged in this space on the HIQ Map, then we would have the healthiest population in the world, a population who took responsibility for their health, their happiness, celebrated what their body can do, and ate sustainably. It really isn't all that far off, and in order for us to get there, we have to do it for ourselves first. People talk about saving the planet and sacrificing themselves for it; the way we save the planet is to look after ourselves first. You cannot pour from an empty cup and you cannot teach what you don't know.

There are four levels of knowing that can play into this and the HIQ Map. These four levels show us the development through the stages of learning right through to embodiment. They have a correlation across to the conscious competence scale as well as the grading scale and HIQ Map.

Those four levels are as follows:

1. Know about
2. Know of
3. Relate to
4. Embody

If you are wanting to master something, then knowing something cognitively isn't enough. To truly have knowledge we must move to embodiment. This is where all of us have knowledge about the subject at hand. Rather than simply knowing cognitively how to do something, we are able to know all the intricacies and possibilities of any given subject or skill. Like the other models, it takes time to move through the levels of knowing and hours of conscious practice. Throughout the book you will have an opportunity to learn which practices will help you with where you are at and to go about practicing them. This is the way we develop any skill. We practice, consciously and deliberately.

Let's use powerlifting as an example in the levels of the knowing scale. When we are at the know-about stage, we can give a rough explanation of what powerlifting is. We may know that it is a strength sport but not be too sure what exercises are involved or how a competition is run. We may know someone who does it or someone whose partner does it. If we talk about the total weight lifted with people here, it won't make much sense as they don't have anything that they personally can compare it to. Anyone at this level won't be able to tell you much more than that, although some of them may try. Although someone at this level will clearly know more than someone who has never heard of it.

Somebody who is at the know-about stage when it comes to powerlifting will be able to tell you that the sport involves three lifts: the bench press, the squat, and the dead lift. They can tell you how the competition is run and even what the goal of the competition is. They may even know about the rules and be familiar with what lifts are regarded as heavy lifts when it comes to total weight lifted. They themselves don't compete or train in this discipline, or if they do, they are in the early stages and are beginning the transition from knowing about to relating with.

To relate to something, we must move past cognitively knowing it and start to use our bodies and senses to connect to it. We must learn what it feels like, what it sounds like, looks like, and experience powerlifting in the mind and body. We must have some type of experience with the sport to be able to really relate to it. This takes time and effort to know what it feels like to complete the lifts, to follow countless programs, and do training sessions even when you don't feel like it, to know what it feels like to fail a lift, to compete on a platform, to lose all motivation. To relate to it we must have a relationship with it. We cannot have a relationship with it without going through the ups and downs of training, lifting, injuries, and the feeling and exhilaration from hitting PRs and overcoming the challenge that powerlifting offers. Although we can talk and talk about powerlifting, even be able to write out a program, powerlifting is something we do; it isn't all that we do. We spend five to ten hours a week training and researching, but it isn't the main thing we do with our time and attention. If you took powerlifting out of our week, even though we may miss it dearly, most of our week would stay the same.

When we embody powerlifting, we live and breathe it. We spend the majority of our week training, teaching, researching, watching, thinking, and even dreaming about powerlifting. Although we do other things, if we took powerlifting and powerlifting related things out of our week you would leave a gaping hole. We have invested blood, sweat, and years of experience in powerlifting, and we may not even compete anymore. However, it is so ingrained in our being that we can close our eyes and vividly imagine what it feels, smells, and looks like to powerlift. We can tell you all the tricks and strategies to cutting weight; we often know the unknowable components to it such as how to mentally prepare for a meet, when to know to stop training to avoid injury due to fatigue, and when to push through. When we embody something to this level, we truly begin to master it, and in this case we wouldn't see powerlifting as a sport. We would see it as a vehicle for a better world, a vehicle that brings people from different backgrounds together to create a community of support, encouragement, and love and as a group overcome their own challenges under the name of powerlifting.

When we embody something, we start to see a deeper meaning behind whatever it is that we have embodied. Powerlifting is no longer just powerlifting. Music is no longer just music. Building a house is no longer just building a house. It moves into an art form with a deeper purpose and meaning. Powerlifting turns into a family of people supporting growth and change. Music turns into a powerful form of communication where people speak from the soul and breathe hope for a better future. A house is turned into a home that is meticulously engineered to be a place of family memories and love.

When we embody our HIQ, it is no longer about being fit and strong. It is about legacy and experience. It is about living and dying. It is about being able to participate in life and juice it for all the juice there is. The dying part often catches people off guard, but it is integral to living. Those who are more aware of their own mortality do not pretend like it won't happen. They don't put off tomorrow what could be done today. They make decisions knowing that one day they won't be here. When we accept our mortality, we choose to live. When we are asleep to that truth, we often stay asleep and wait. The embodiment of our health allows us to wake up to life and live the life we so truly want while building a legacy and a path for those who follow us.

To conclude this chapter, I want to emphasize the importance of using the HIQ Map for yourself and using it to deepen your understanding of yourself. The result of doing that allows you to experience life on a richer level and know just what you need to do in order to squeeze the most out of life itself.

PART I

The
MIND

Living the Dream

In order to live our dream, we must first get rid of the bullshit that's holding us back and identify what our dream actually is. Sometimes we over complicate our dreams. We dream of a big home, lots of money, mojitos on the beach, but they aren't really our dreams. Those are often disguised as the need to feel important, to have security, and to not feel guilty about relaxing.

If you have a big home that's empty, is that your dream? Or is it a reflection of how you feel? If you have lots of money but more debt and no real human connections, is that also your dream? Or is it now a fear? At some point the mojitos will get old and life will become meaningless. What do you do then?

Often people mistake their goals for ideals. They set goals based on what they think will give them what they want. Not on what they actually want.

Tony Robbins preaches the six core human needs as a means of understanding what we humans are really seeking. This is strikingly different to Maslow's Hierarchy of needs. The six core needs can help us gain a clearer understanding of what is the motivation behind our goals. To deepen our understating of why we want what we want can increase the likelihood of achieving the goal. People can be guilty of getting upset over goals they didn't really want and fail to get because it reinforces a deep seeded belief of them being faulty and absent of the ability to see things through to the end. They didn't want the goal, which is probably why they didn't get it, but then it also strengthens a limiting belief they have of themselves and drives them further away from their true goal as it strengthens the thoughts that tell them they don't deserve it. We don't get what we want; we get what we are willing to receive and what we think we deserve.

Understanding the six core needs can help us strengthen our why, and in some cases even realize that what we say we want isn't really what we want and then change course accordingly.

The six core human needs that we seek to fulfill are the following:

Personality Needs

Certainty

• The need for safety, security, comfort, order, consistency.

Uncertainty or Variety

• The need for change, surprise, the unknown, challenge, excitement.

Significance

• The need to feel important, to have meaning, sense of self, worthiness of love.

Love or Connection

- The need to be a part of something, to be accepted, to feel wanted, to feel loved by and cared for.

Spiritual Needs

Contribution

- The need to give back, to care for, to deepen meaning, leave a legacy, protect, and serve.

Growth

- The need for continual improvement and development of the mind, body, and spirit.

The first four of the needs are personality needs, and the last two are spiritual needs. When broken down, every goal we have falls under one of the above categories. They may be communicated slightly differently; for example, someone may say they want to be accepted rather than stating they want to feel connected. Knowing this is crucial for us to not only set worthy goals but to also deeply understand why it is important to us and, conversely, if it isn't important to us.

A good example of this would be somebody wanting to start a business. Let's use the fitness industry as the example. They set out wanting to start a gym and making a positive impact in people's lives. The reason behind this goal could be the following:

Certainty: to have control over their life and be in charge of making decisions on their future

Variety: to have a new challenge in life or to do different things each day and deal with a whole new group of people

Significance: to prove someone wrong or to try and get their approval, an attempt to feel important as an owner rather than as a personal trainer

Connection: to build a community based on their own values and have a family outside of their immediate family

Contribution: to make a bigger impact on the world and leave a legacy

Growth: to take the next step in their career and continually be in a place where they either sink or swim

If we simply understand the goal on the superficial objective level, then we can miss the deeper reason why we are pursuing it. We pursue a goal because we believe it will give us something we don't currently have.

If we take weight loss as the example again, we start to see how even though people may lose weight, if they don't also achieve what they truly want, then they still won't be happy.

Here are some examples as to why somebody may want to lose weight:

Certainty: to take control of their health after a toxic relationship where they felt out of control

Variety: to start participating more in life so that they can experience the moments that they feel they are missing out on by sitting on the sidelines.

Significance: to feel attractive and confident, to take care of themselves as if they were someone worth taking care of, that is to be significant to themselves

Connection: be healthy enough to play with their children and build memories for life

Contribution: to be an example and show the world you can turn your life around

Growth: to understand themselves more and to experience more in life through their body that they were gifted

If someone was just to lose weight yet wasn't able to connect to the deeper reason, then we may find that the result will only be fleeting. Nothing has changed. Nothing has been achieved. The person is still in the same place as they were before, just with a new wardrobe, one that they will have to sell or throw out if the results go back to where they were before they started the fitness journey, which is so often the case.

As you can see in the above example, if the person doesn't have a worthy pursuit and continually develops their HIQ through education and love, then they yo-yo. They look for superficial goals and are provided with superficial solutions. So many people are afraid to go deep but that is where you experience life. It is also where you can complicate life, but at its core, it is where we can truly understand ourselves and experience the richness that life has to offer. If we live superficially, then our experience is also superficial. People aren't afraid of love, they are afraid of not being loved in return. They are afraid of being rejected because they have rejected themselves. So they live superficially and keep people at arm's length in order to protect themselves from pain, not realizing that they are constantly in it.

One important question we can ask ourselves is, what key experiences do we want to have in this life? When we set experience-based goals, we challenge ourselves to gain something in the form of a memory or a way of contributing and giving back that which helps deepen the connection we have to achieving our goal. What is the experience we want to gain from losing 20 kg? What is the experience we wish to gain from starting our own business? What is the experience we wish to gain from starting a family or buying a home?

When we get to the experience and see what that will give us that we don't already have, then that is one sure way to truly connect to our goals and build a strong bond with the sense of achieving them.

Goals vs. Resolutions

Sometimes people don't reach their goals because they aren't goals but resolutions. In essence, a resolution is something you continually work toward and do, whereas a goal is specific and has a predetermined completion date. A resolution is a promise to yourself and is often made up by a cluster of goals. There are a number of different ways people want to describe the differences, but the key thing is that they are different.

A New Year's resolution like "losing 10 kg" or "running a marathon" is a goal, not a resolution. A resolution is to train five days a week for twelve weeks. The word "resolution" comes from the word "resolute," which is to be admirably purposeful, determined, and unwavering. When we bring energy and determination to our goals, we give ourselves the best chance of success. Being resolute about going to the gym five days a week will give us the best chance of running a marathon or anything else we are training for.

A resolution is more likened to the habits and behaviors we wish to develop continually; a goal is something finite and measurable. This is why we are asked about our New Year's resolutions. We aren't being asked what we want to achieve, we are being asked who we want to become and what habits we want to build in order to become that person. Goals and resolutions go hand in hand to give us the best chance of success for our dreams and in life.

The Different Ways to Set Goals

S.M.A.R.T Goals

One of the ways to address our goals is through the SMART method—setting goals that are Specific, Measurable, Achievable, Realistic (or Relative), and Timely. This is possibly the most renowned approach when it comes to goals and although I don't personally use it, it would be ignorant to think that this system doesn't provide value and hasn't worked for people in the past. If this is your preferred method of setting goals, then by all means use it.

There are two main reasons why I don't personally use SMART goals. The first issue I have with SMART goals is with the achievable component of SMART. This encourages us to only set goals that are conceived to be achievable and in the eyes of whom? In my eyes, it presupposes to only set goals based on the knowledge you have now and lacks the foresight to change the future. So many inventions would have died on the conveyer belt of SMART goals as they were often seen as impossible. The second issue is with the realistic component. Once again, a lot of inventions and goals would have died here as so many goals would have been seen as unrealistic and impossible to achieve. One of the factors that can work in the favor of SMART goals is that at the core you have to believe that the goals you are setting are realistic and achievable and hold that unwavering belief even if no one else can see what you can see and no matter what anyone else says. This in itself is not bad advice when it comes to setting targets for your life.

My personal opinion aside, SMART goals can and do work. The only thing to add to your goals would be the format in which you wish to set them, for example, putting 15 to 20 minutes aside on each area of your life.

Zig Ziglar has developed the wheel of life, which offers seven areas to set goals in, they are the following:

1. Personal, social, and recreation
   - Goals revolving around what you like to do for fun, who you spend your time with, and things you spend free time doing like hobbies

2. Work, business, or career
   - Goals revolving around your life's work, what you want to do for a job, or where you want your business to be in a year's time, or even changing careers

3. Family and romantic relationships
   - Goals revolving around your relationship with your spouse, family holidays, and traditions, future family members, or even future spouses

4. Spiritual
   - Goals revolving around being connected to the spiritual side of you, to deepen the connection you have with your true essence and being

5. Financial
   - Goals revolving around income and other revenue sources, budgeting and cutting unnecessary costs

6. Mind and personal development
   - Goals revolving around learning and developing the skill set of your mind, learning strategies to strengthen your mental game

7. Physical fitness and health
   - Goals revolving around your body and physical capabilities, could be sporting events, a new training program or personal physical goals

The 135FOUR Goals

135FOUR (read one, three, five, four) goals was my rebuttal to the SMART-goal phenomenon. In retrospect, you can even use the SMART method to go over your finished goals and check to make sure they are specific, measurable, achievable, relatable, and have a time frame. The 135FOUR method helps to prioritize your goals, plan them out, and build a push/pull motivation toward what we do want and away from what we don't.

One of the challenges that the 135FOUR method brings is that you have to get personal and dig deep. This does not work well if you have global and superficial answers to the questions. We want to have a deeper meaning and an emotionally compelling why behind your goals.

If you are able to put yourself in a place of pure honesty and vulnerability, then the 135FOUR method can help you pinpoint your goal, why you want it, and how to take your first steps.

You can use this formula for planning out the decade, the year, the month, or even the day. I recommend using it to set long-term goals (1 to 10-plus years) and short-term goals (less than 12 months).

I recommend using the seven areas that were mentioned before and setting a timer for ten minutes per area. During the five to ten minutes, write down as many goals that come to you as possible. Don't worry about getting them right or seeing them and laughing and making you clean the toilet or anything silly. Just write whatever comes up; you can delete those ones later that aren't a fit for you.

Once you have done that for each area, go over it and mark an asterisk next to the three most important goals in each area. This will in turn give you a total of 21 goals to make your list from. Don't worry if it is a little bit less or if you find it challenging to cut them down to only 21. Each person will have their own challenge; don't get stuck on the details. There is no right way to goal set, but there is a wrong way, and the wrong way is to not complete it.

Now we have a list of goals to use for our 135FOUR goal-setting format.

In this format the goals are set out in three different categories. There is one A goal, three B goals, and five C goals. The A goal is by far the most important and meaningful; if it was achieved, it could make the rest either obsolete or complete. This could be something like starting a dream business, studying a subject you have always wanted, or buying a family home.

The B goals may support the A goal. A B goal isn't something that you are able to just go and either purchase or do; it is something that is still important and will take a period of time to do but not quite as important or meaningful as the A1 goal. Some examples of B goals could be finding a business mentor and signing up to a six-month course, purchasing and reading six books on owning my first property, or being fit enough to be competitive in an obstacle course race in a year's time.

The C goals are the smaller often more fun goals and can sometimes be seen as not important. These goals, however, can be argued to be the most important. The other goals can often take time, and if we aren't careful, we could lose momentum and motivation. The C goals allow us to tick things off as we go. They can either be in aid of the B and A goals or can be completely independent. These can be goals like sky diving, booking a holiday, or asking someone on a date. Maybe that last one is a little scarier than sky diving, but both can be done in a short period of time.

135FOUR

The 1 in 135 stands for your A1 goal. This is the goal that if achieved would make everything else either complete or redundant. It is your keystone goal, where if you were to achieve one thing and nothing else, what would you choose? It is the goal with the most purpose and depth to it. This goal should scare you and stretch you beyond what is comfortable. You should have to grow as a person to reach this goal. You would have to grow to a level you are not at yet. When setting this goal, it is important to not be restricted to the resources that you currently have. Setting it on resources you don't have yet can help inspire you to find ways to make it happen.

The 3 stands for your B1, B2, B3 goals. These are secondary goals. Goals that will be challenging yet achievable for you. These goals can often help support and lead you to your A1 goal. They can also stand alone and represent personal development and pursuit of growth.

The 5 stands for your C1, C2, C3, C4, C5 goals. These goals are all preliminary goals or low-hanging fruit. They are usually fun and challenging and things that you have been putting off. Just because these goals aren't massive purpose-driven goals doesn't mean they aren't important. Little wins help set up the big wins. The more little wins we can do, the more we gain momentum for the big ones. These can often be simple goals like, learn to surf, read a book a month, or call Mum every Tuesday.

Now that you have approximately 21 goals to choose from, start placing them in the 135 goal format. If you are unsure where something should go, if it is more important than another goal, ask yourself, if you could have one but not the other, which one you would choose. This doesn't mean you eliminate the other goal, it is just to help shape your goal hierarchy.

Once you have a goal for each 1, 3, and 5 slot, it is time to move on to the big FOUR.

The FOUR stands for the big four questions we ask ourselves to help support the goals and set a plan. It is important that we access both head and heart when setting goals as logical goals will fall by the wayside when we feel deflated, and emotional goals can often go unstructured especially if they lack a plan.

Once you have completed your 135, go through each question and ask,

When is this to be completed? (logical)

- The importance of this question is to have an end date so that you have a target to aim for. This will help push you each day, knowing well that the date is getting closer and closer. It helps keep you accountable and the goal on top of your mind. Sometimes we may not know be able to tell when it will be completed, but what we can do is select a date so that the first task on the way to completing that goal can be completed. When choosing a completion date, it is important to make sure you have a realistic time frame to complete the goal. Ensure that you have looked at all impeding factors that may stall your goal and be firm but flexible when it comes to the target date. Life happens; it is better to achieve it later than not to achieve it at all.

Why is this important to me? (emotional)

- Your why is your pull. It should be emotional, inspiring, and compelling. Often our first response to this question can kind of feel a bit shallow and awkward. That's okay, keep trying. This helps the goal to be purpose driven and gives it a deep meaning providing conviction. Some questions that can help with writing out your why are the following:

» What will I gain from this that I don't already have?
» How will this change my life?
» What makes me drawn to achieving this goal?
» Who else does this goal positively impact?

It is so crucial to be brutally honest with ourselves here no matter how silly it sounds or we think it may sound to someone else. These goals are for us to achieve, and understanding the why and making a deep connection to achieving it will help secure the motivation required to obtaining your goal. Go deep and get connected to the goal.

How do I see this goal being completed? (logical)

• This is where we start to plan your goal out. If you can see your goal step by step, then write it step by step. If you don't know your goal step by step yet, then set the first step and make sure it is an action step with an actionable date, objective, and someone to be accountable to. We don't need to know all the steps and stages, they often appear on the way. Even if we do know all the steps and stages, there are so many changing factors that they are likely to change over time. As with all the questions, the more description here the better. Don't get hung up on knowing all the steps, set out what is important and figure out the first step. There is a Rumi quote that fits beautifully here: "As you start to walk on the way, the way appears."

What happens if you don't? (emotional)

- What happens if you don't achieve your goal? What pain will you experience? Whom will you let down? What is the real cost of you failing to meet this goal? What will that mean for you? What will it cost you financially, emotionally, in your relationships or with yourself? This is your push and motivation. More people are motivated by pain than by the idea of pleasure. Get deep here; it will pay off. The key thing here is to build a compelling target to aim toward and having a painful association with a situation or circumstance to move away from.

Here is the 135FOUR template for you to fill out.

A1:

What?

When?

Why?

How?

What if?

B1:

What?

When?

Why?

How?

What if?

B2:

What?

When?

Why?

How?

What if?

B3:

What?

When?

Why?

How?

What if?

C1:

What?

When?

Why?

How?

What if?

C2:

What?

When?

Why?

How?

What if?

C3:

What?

When?

Why?

How?

What if?

C4:

What?

When?

Why?

How?

What if?

C5:

What?

When?

Why?

How?

What if?

Goals and the HIQ Map

The HIQ Map works in conjunction to your overarching goal. Once you have your goal in place, you use the HIQ Map to measure where you need to be in order to achieve that goal. Because our goals can change throughout life and make different demands of our time and energy, the map can be used by any one at any time to help them better understand what is required of them to best put them in a position to achieve their goal.

For example, one year a woman has a goal to lose 20 kg and gain her freedom back, the next year she wants to run a half marathon, and then the following year she wants to have her first child, then she will likely need different nutritional plans, training programs, a strong mind-body connection through the different life and body changes she will undergo. Her overarching goal will change over those three years and so will her nutritional needs, her physical needs, her recovery needs, and not to mention all the unknowns that go into those three different life situations.

Sometimes the overarching goal is to finish a master's degree or start a business; if this is the case, then HIQ can play a role to help people best get an understanding of where they can drop down to under times of stress and where they can make the healthiest choices to keep their baseline HIQ as high as possible. Other times, it can just be used to gauge the gap of where we are and where we want to be in order to live our best life. Sometimes people aren't really certain what their goal is and will often find out their goal by trying a bunch of things. You don't always have to have the perfect goal to get started; sometimes getting started is the goal and that is good enough. There is no perfect goal, there is no perfect time to start, which, ironically, means every time and every goal is therefore perfect. Another way to think about it is that you don't have to be great to start, but you have to start to be great.

Once you have penned your A1 or your smartest of SMART goals, use the next three chapters to establish your baseline within the three areas that make up HIQ and recognize which stage is best suited to execute your goal or goals. It is normal to have different levels and stages as we all have areas we are more comfortable with and stronger with. Remember this is identifying the areas we can improve on to live our best life outside of the gym. There is no good or bad or right or wrong, just where we are, where we want to be, and the necessary steps to take on our way to achieving our goals.

The Mind Is Primary

"You have work to do."

These were Rob McDonald's words to me post my first workout at the infamous Gym Jones in Salt Lake City. At the time of this writing, Rob and Gym Jones are no longer connected, but both Gym Jones and Rob McDonald have played roles in me understanding myself and training better.

The gym itself maybe 250 square meters with some other rooms coming off the main floor, a couple of racks, about six rowers, four SkiErgs, four AirBikes, some boxes, a boxing bag, and then there's you.

Gym Jones was my first inspiration when it came to functional training. I remember seeing Mark Twight's YouTube video of him training the actors of *300*. That was what changed training for me. That's where it all started.

Although I don't think Gym Jones got everything right, they definitely got one thing right; the mind is primary.

From here on, when I talk about Gym Jones in this book, it could go on to mean a number of people. I am going to use the term broadly to mean the facility and anyone involved with it at the time of my experience with it.

Gym Jones understood the connection the mind has with the body and its ability to push the limits of the mind in order to push the body and vice versa. It knew the mind would give up before the body would. It is a survival tactic. Your mind is attempting to keep energy for a later threat in an attempt to protect you. Makes sense.

This chapter and section of the book is really about truly understanding ourselves, what drives our motivations, and how to train ourselves mentally to get the most out of our lives. Our mental health is integral to our overall health, and it is often ignored as if it just is or isn't. We don't just happen to be physically fit or not physically fit. We still have to exercise and rest and learn more about our bodies in order to become physically fit. Our mental health is exactly the same. We need to train our mind and practice so that we are able to continually stay mentally fit and healthy. Often we just accept ourselves as we are and then assume that is our mental health and how it is always going to be. This static view of mental health is not only incorrect, but it is potentially dangerous. One of the best ways to view the mind is to see it as a forever unfolding and dynamic process like a movie rather than a photo. In this book, when I refer to the mind, I am referring to an integration of the thoughts we hold in mind, our spirit, or as I will call it, our essence, and our emotions and felt experiences. Our society has put such high value on physical fitness and physical health, and only in very recent times have we started to shed light on the importance of taking care of our mental health.

For the large majority of the population we are able to use mental practices, education, physical exercise, and nutrition to ensure that our mental health is strong and robust. This section of the book will offer suggestions on learning and awareness to further understand our own minds and best practices for continual improvement.

Like Gym Jones, I see the mind as being primary to all our goals as well as playing a role in each area of our HIQ. It is crucial to truly understand one thing: when it comes to developing our mind there is no finish line. As soon as we think we have it all figured out, the further away we seem to be from doing just that. The mind is not to be conquered; it is to be understood, to be accepted.

The HIQ Mind Map

So when it comes to developing our mental game, what's the outcome? What's the end goal?

These are great questions. And questions I don't have the answer to. Nor should I. The end goal is going to be different for each person. We are going to develop at different rates. What you think is the end goal for you today will ultimately amend its self naturally as you mature and age. My guess is that you have gained an incredible amount of insight and have gone through an incredible amount of lessons over the past 10 years, which have altered the way you look at the world. What makes you think that that's not going to happen again? Look around you, everything is temporary.

Everything.

And that's okay.

We are on this planet for a little while. It is selfless to pursue our potential, to learn about ourselves so that we can be kind to ourselves and teach others to be kind to us. When we are kind to ourselves, we can be truly connected and kind to others.

The whole idea is transcendence of where we are now. Not just a six-pack, not just a weight goal. And no, not even to fit into those jeans. None of those things have anything to do with our true self-worth and happiness. This doesn't mean we shouldn't obtain or achieve them; it means that these things are possible by-products of what is important to us.

The goal is to end unnecessary suffering. It was Seneca who said we suffer more in our imagination than we do in reality. I remember one time I was on a podcast in a gym in Salt Lake City, and the guys asked what my end goal was. I told them it was to get rid of all preventable mental health issues. They laughed.

The key word there is "preventable." It is all that is unnecessary. So we have to ask ourselves, is the suffering I am going through necessary? And sometimes it is. Sometimes it is what we need. We don't get the goals we ask for; we get the problems we need to solve in order to achieve our goals. Most people stop here, thinking the world didn't get them what they wanted. Often your problems are exactly what you asked for.

So what about suffering? Isn't a little suffering a good thing? Can't some stress be healthy? Yes. I would go even as far to say that I used to think suffering was what the weak did; now I understand it is what the weak avoid as if we aren't allowed to suffer a little bit be it physical, emotional, or mental. The suffering can sometimes be the rent we have to pay in order to mature into the person we deserve to be.

It is the unnecessary suffering we must build immunity to. Because hurt people hurt people. When we look after ourselves and take care of our own hurt, we unintentionally inspire others to do the same.

The game is in the mind. It shapes your reality. But like physical training, it has to be sharpened and looked after every day. People say you are the average of the five people you hang around; what they don't talk about is working on yourself to be the kind of person people want to be around.

You have to define what's your end goal? How much are you going to commit to training your mind? Training your thoughts? To take ruthless responsibility of your own emotions? We often have to let go of who we are now in order to become who we deserve to be in order to step into our potential. Who could you be if you acted in accordance to your potential today?

The Three Stages of the HIQ Mind Map

The idea behind the three stages of the HIQ is to figure out what you want in life and then where you need to be in order to live that life. The same goes for the mind as it does for movement and nutrition.

The three stages of the HIQ Mind Map are the following:

- Student
- Scholar
- Sage

When it comes to the mind side of things, the goal isn't necessarily to transcend to the highest level of being to become the all-knowing, all-seeing almighty being of beings. It is to simply recognize where you are on your path and to then figure out what you need to do next to move closer to where you want to be. Sometimes it isn't even about needing to know where you want to be. It can just be about being okay with the process as it unfolds.

The goal of understanding the student, scholar, and sage stages of this chapter is to grasp what the stages are, what the paths of development are, and what other resources may be of benefit to you. There isn't just one book that will be able teach you everything you need to know. This book is simply just one resource in an abundance of resources. The other books that I have mentioned so far are more resources that can benefit you on understanding yourself on a deeper level, as can many more books and authors that I also mention throughout the book. Some of the books you may have already read, and some of the content I speak of you may have already read. Since no man or woman steps into the same river twice, it may be worth going back and rereading them with a new lens of life. You may find lessons that were there the whole time. Life is after all a learning process. There is no finish line, and you aren't supposed to arrive anywhere by any time. You have the opportunity to continually learn in every single moment. Whether we do or not is up to us.

The difficulty a lot of people have with this area of content is how subjective it is. It is challenging to define specifically where someone may be, and because of that a lot of people who really lean into objectivity will struggle with this component. An easy way to think about the objective and subjective benefits and the difficulty of measuring the subjective is when we consider a job.

When we apply for a job, it will have particular roles expected, benefits, and of course the starting salary. When we apply for a job, the salary plays a role in what we apply for. Fair enough too because, you know, money is pretty useful. The good thing when it comes to money is that it is easy to measure. We can compare jobs based on income. For the sake of this example, let's say they are earning good old Australian Dollars. Or Dollarydoos for anyone who watched *The Simpsons*. If one job is paying $50K per annum and the other job is paying $70K per annum, then which one would you pick? Possibly the $70K, unless you have more questions such as, what are the hours? What is the culture of the business like? What about if one job was $50K and the other was $120K? It may sway your decision further.

An important question here is how happy will you be in that job? How happy is happy? What conditions in the business will make you happy? How do you measure happiness? We all know how important it is, but yet there isn't an obvious universal measurement that we all use. The metric system doesn't have one. Nor does the imperial. But we know it is important. What about unhappiness? How do we measure that? It isn't as obvious as salary.

That is because happiness is subjective. You can't point at it. You can't put it in a wheelbarrow. Happiness occurs in the mind. People may say you can point at a smile or you can put a puppy in a wheelbarrow. But those things aren't happiness. A smile is a muscular reaction we sometimes have toward things that may make us happy, but not always, and, well, a puppy is a pretty good symbol of happiness, but it is what the puppy means to us that makes us happy. Meanings don't go into wheelbarrows; they are in our mind.

So then you have to ask, how long can you put up with a bad culture, tyrannical boss, and 60-hour weeks for an extra $70K? Will you really quit after one year like you said you would? Or would the money give you too much "freedom." Is an extra $70K a year worth being unhappy for? How much can someone pay you to miss your daughter's recital? How much can someone pay you to travel 100 days a year and live apart from your spouse? How much can someone pay us to be unhappy? The sad thing to face is that most people's salaries are just hush money for their dreams.

This whole chapter isn't looking at your salary. It is looking at your mental environment and mapping. It is looking at how much self-work we do to ensure that we have a high happiness salary. That part is up to us. It is up to our choices. What's interesting is that some people mistake happiness for excitement. Excitement is about the future. True happiness is peacefulness. It is being at peace with the present. Excitement is about what is to come, it is not about what is now. It is not true happiness.

There is of course more to life than just happiness. Although a noble quest, purpose, and meaning among other values come into play, the point of sharing all the content on happiness was to express the fact that not everything in life that is important is easy to measure. It wasn't to overvalue happiness. When things are subjective, they become harder to measure. That doesn't mean there aren't measurements or that we should just give up on it. What it does mean is that in the Western world we haven't traditionally put a lot of value on things we can't measure. Hence you can measure the salary, but it's a little harder (not impossible) to measure the culture of a workplace.

So how do we measure the coming chapters then? Great question. We will mostly be using the conscious competence scale described in an earlier chapter and integrating that with the levels of healthiness of the Enneagram.

For those who are interested in extra reading, I would recommend learning about the Development Stages of Consciousness by Ken Wilber. *A Brief History of Everything* is a good place to start. Another book on a similar subject is *Spiral Dynamics* by Chris Cowan and Don Beck. The concept of spiral dynamics was initially developed by Clare Graves and is one of the components integrated into Ken's Development Stages of Consciousness.

Now that we have covered all that, where do you sit on the levels of the HIQ Mind Map?

Student

The first thing we want to understand is the three main areas of the mind map, what each area involves, and paths of development. Each stage comes with recommended standards to meet to reach that stage. One of the important things to remember is that this whole map is just a guide. So although the standards and what I offer throughout this book has been well researched and implemented with success, it is really up to you to decide what's important for you, what is worth implementing, and what will fit into your life. The importance of recognizing where we may fit into the model allows us to see where we are. Of course this means we know where we are starting from, but most importantly it means we are able to recognize what is the first step. What is the one thing that I could do that I would do? As I have repeated multiple times throughout this book, your life is one big unfolding process. Like any map, if we are wanting to get from one place to the other, we cannot skip going through all the towns along the way. This means that if we want to go from Los Angeles to New York, we have to cross the whole country. Of course to follow the analogy, you can walk, drive, or even fly between these two locations. Or you could even go totally the wrong way. So many people are sitting in Los Angeles talking about how they want to go to New York but just expecting it to happen without the work. My biggest offer is to have an open mind and try new points of view. If we want different results, we need to have different thinking in order to get there.

The first level of the HIQ Mind Map is the student level. At this early stage, we first start taking responsibility for learning more about ourselves. This when we first begin to start to become aware of our thoughts and realize that we may want a different result from what we are currently getting in one or more areas of our lives. Because of this, we start to become a student of life but, like when we start school, we aren't aware of just how much we don't know. If you were to compare this to the conscious competency scale, this would be the conscious incompetence stage. We are aware that there is so much we don't yet know, and some of it doesn't even make sense yet, and we may be unsure if it ever will. Everything we learn and read is brand new. It may have been there before (hint: it always was), but we never heard it, never saw it, and didn't care for it.

All of a sudden, things start making more sense, and we start gaining more curiosity. This is the first stage in taking responsibility for our own emotions and thoughts. The student stage of development is a pivotal moment in one's life. It is when one stops tolerating being treated in a particular way and starts to stand up for oneself. Sadly, some people never make it to this initial stage. They stay in their unconscious incompetence stage and will continue to play victim to the world. They will go round and round in drama cycles and codependent relationships while blaming the world for their shortcomings.

Students at this level start to realize they have a choice. They can choose to wallow, or they can choose to do something about it. So they choose to do something. A lot of people can be scared to start because they don't know where to start. It doesn't matter where you start, and never be afraid of making mistakes. When you start, you will naturally make mistakes. Even the word "mistake" means missed take. You took the opportunity, you just missed. Go again! And when we step back and really look at it, those weren't mistakes, they were lessons. They were the assignments for us to learn how to get what we want.

Often when you start, you may find yourself going down a couple of dead ends—some books that don't really hit home, a seminar that seemed way too woo woo! And way, and I mean way, too many people trying to sell you oils, shakes, and supplements #bossbabe. That is all part of the process. Maybe your process may sound different to that, and that's completely fine. What's important is that you start your student journey of self-learning. The goal of this chapter is to point you in a direction for you to continue down your path as a student, to help you identify whereabouts you sit with regard to the mind component of the HIQ Map, and to offer ways to continue your personal development.

Signs of This Developmental Stage
Some key signs of this stage are

- becoming increasingly curious about life and ways to develop;
- a continual desire to share learnings straight away;
- a new lease of life;
- intellectual understanding of the principles learned, but yet to embody them;
- possible struggle to let go of old patterns and relationships;
- searching for new groups and people;

- the possibility of dropping back down to a static substudent stage, which is a static stage of understanding there is something there to work on, but too busy in life to do so. It is like walking on top of a subway. There is something down there that can take me to where I want to go but I am too busy up here doing day-to-day tasks;
- excitement about new gains, whether they be knowledge gains or physical gains from training; and
- a possible level of embarrassment that comes with finding out all this new information as if the student should have known this all before.

It is important to note that this stage is different to development for work purposes. This is development of self. Some people have developed skills for their workplace and that's where it stays. They do courses, read books to further their career, and never carry it over to their actual life outside of work, to their relationships with their spouse, their kids, family, and, most importantly, to themselves. People don't have problems in their careers, they have personal problems that flow into their careers. I have worked with countless professionals who were emotionally and personally lost. They were so good at developing their skills for their job that they almost used it as an escape from facing and developing themselves. You can be a 50-year-old professional and just coming on as a student here. There is nothing wrong with that; it unfolds as it does. There is no wasted time; there is only life.

Student Benchmarks

These benchmarks are measured yearly and are very attainable. Long term, these small changes can change your life. If you are to think of one person who makes zero changes compared to the person who makes these changes and fast-forward 10 years, you will find there is a large gap between where they start and where they find themselves a decade later. This is evidence of small steps that make up large leaps.

The student benchmarks are as follows:

* **Six Books/E-books per Year**

  In our busy world, we often neglect the importance of reading biographies, books on personal development, novels, and best-selling how-to books. Luckily for us, we live in a time where we can simply order these books online, and they rock up to our home in just a few short days. If you are completely time poor, you can even download them on an app as an e-book. If you are even more time poor, you can even speed up the e-book on most apps so that you can complete them twice as fast. You can listen to them when you're making dinner, getting ready in the morning, or driving to work. It can literally almost take no effort to enable you to digest books. Your brain is extremely complex and can take in bucketloads of information subconsciously, so even if you aren't taking notes, your brain definitely is.

* **Two Weekend Training Courses or Equivalent**

One of the benefits of attending training courses biannually is to not only learn the content that they teach but to also get around like-minded people. One of the hardest things when making a transition into being a student of life is momentum. Being around people going the same way as you can make a massive difference to whether you continue down that path or not. Two training courses a year could either be equivalent to two or four days a year. That still leaves you with 361 days in a year to do everything else you need to do. Invest in yourself.

- **Twenty-Five Hours of Mood Prep/Quiet Time per Year**

Putting time aside for ourselves and to quiet our minds can appear to be near impossible for some of us, especially parents. Often the best time to do this is first thing in the morning before the rest of the world catches up with us. Five minutes, six days a week, for 52 weeks a year equates to 26 hours a year. Five minutes can be all you need to help prep your mood and keep you sane. Although it doesn't appear to be much, 260 hours over 10 years is arguably a better practice than scrolling social media for that amount of time.

I even started a 10-minute podcast Monday to Friday titled *Mood Prep* to give people an opportunity to consume something mentally stimulating and help people prep their mood for the day. The podcast covers psychology, stoic philosophy, Neuro-Linguistic Programming (or NLP), coaching, behavioral psychology subjects, and basic tips to start the day on the right foot. In my early 20s, when I started to really struggle with my business and struggle personally, I would get up and listen to something positive and motivating first thing in the morning to help set me for the day and get me in the right mood to tackle the challenges. *Mood Prep* is designed for people to do just that.

Scholar

The only way we can truly develop from student to scholar is through time and application. In this stage we really start to not just know about the types of personal development on offer but also know about them and truly relate to them. During this stage it becomes a part of our daily practice, and the main difference between this and the student level is experience. A lot of mistakes and failures have led to breakthroughs and aha moments. People at this stage understand that they never leave the student level. They transcend and include it. They are still students of life; they just have a bucket load more experience behind them that gives them depth and self-awareness they didn't previously have. Metaphorically speaking these people are either just finishing university or college of life and are truly learning to embody their learnings in the real world, not just in their head. They aren't satisfied with just "knowing"; they want to truly embody their learnings. At later stages, they start to teach their learnings. They do so in a way very different to those in the student level, who just talk to whoever they can about it whether they are interested or not. In the later stages of scholar level, the students start to recognize those who are truly interested and those who aren't. They don't judge those who aren't; they just don't spend unnecessary time justifying themselves or what they have learned to people who aren't interested.

The scholar level is where people really go deep in their own personal learning and understand that it's not about changing the world; it is about changing themselves. They start to really own the concept that if you want to change the world, then you must change your inner world. They understand that it isn't a switch, that things don't just change all of a sudden, and that for things to change the ingredient of time is necessary.

Signs of This Developmental Stage

Some key signs of this stage are that scholars

- begin to truly live their personal principles and understand that everything is fluid and constantly changing;
- share learnings with people who are interested in hearing about them;
- integrate development into their daily life;
- begin embodying some of the principles they have learned over time;
- continually find old patterns and thoughts that no longer serve them and go about clearing these as they move through life;
- are integral members of the groups they belong to;
- many find this to be the stage that they stay with. A large population that move to this stage come to realize that this is enough for what they want to get out of life;
- are at a stage in life where gains are a by-product of them focusing on the process; and
- have likely invested thousands of dollars and possibly hundreds if not thousands of hours on their learning.

Scholar Benchmarks

The scholar benchmarks are as follows:

- **Twelve Books/E-books/Audio Books per Year**

Once you have started the habit of putting time aside for yourself, consuming 1 book a month becomes easier than once thought. For a lot of people, even 1 book a month from the outset may be too many. If we were to continue down the path of consuming just 1 book a month, we read 120 books every 10 years. Imagine what the difference would be if you were to compare the two people, one of whom had consumed 120 books within the last 10 years and the other nil? This isn't to shame the individual who chooses not to read; this is to encourage those of us who have the desire to do so.

- **Four to Eight Weekends of Training Courses or Equivalent**

Eight days a year on personal development still leaves a bucketload more days in the year to get shit done. I have done courses that ran 9:00 a.m.–9:00 p.m. straight for eight days. I highly recommend finding the courses that pique your interest and investing in yourself. Of course, do your homework on which educators you align with the most; either way I highly recommend that if you are wanting to continually delve deeper, then go deep into education. The reality is that some courses may miss the mark; it happens. Don't let that hold you back. Simply by adding in a couple more seminars or courses throughout the year, we help to keep our own development top of mind and move past just being a student of our own life. When we combine this with 12 books a year, we truly have the ability to look at the world and our own life through a completely different lens.

- **Fifty Hours of Mood Prep/Quiet Time per Year**

They say that if you don't have 10 minutes, then you don't have a life. By simply mood prepping for a total of 10 minutes a day you can not only take on the day and its challenges with ease but also build the mental fortitude you need when you get thrown off path or deal with difficult situations. I release a minimum of 250 episodes a year of *Mood Prep*. That by itself is about 42 hours of development. Podcasts and apps like YouTube make it so easy to access quality information, not to mention the apps available for those of us who struggle with things like meditation.

Sage

The sage stage is not to be taken lightly. Ken Wilber talks about high-level thinkers as second tier thinkers. These people think systemically and do large amounts of personal work to clear their own crap. People at this stage are genuine thought leaders and people of action. One of the key things to know about these people is that they don't have to tell you. They live aligned to their purpose and what's pulling them from within. Their self-awareness transcends the physical plane, and they see the integration of the mind, the body, and the heart. They see how things impact globally and are true empathetic leaders. Such a person could be the mother of the family that you live next door to, a political figure, or even a local business owner. They see how everything is connected and understand what is within their power to take responsibility of and lead a noble life.

Often these people get criticized as having their heads in the clouds when really they are just ahead of the bell curve. They have spent years mastering their mind and will continue to pursue their potential and share their findings for the benefit of others. They have grown past the idea of sacrificing self for others and instead develop self for others. The sage stops answering questions to show their wisdom but rather proposes questions to bring out the solution in the person seeking an answer. In doing so they strengthen the other individual's problem-solving skills, confidence in self, and self-awareness. People at lower stages may get annoyed with what appears to be this person's inability to answer questions as they are seeking answers without rather than within. This doesn't mean we don't need answers sometimes; it just means that more often than not, a lot of people know the answers to the questions they are asking; they just want to hear them from an external source. The sage knows that smart people have great answers and wise people have better questions.

Signs of This Developmental Stage

Some key signs of this stage are that sages

- embody the life lessons they have learned and are most likely teaching them in one fashion or another;
- are a source of information and education for those who are seeking it;
- are often teachers, as to teach is to learn twice;
- live the life of someone who is a constant student of life;
- will often work through old frames and limiting beliefs in moments, and people around them wouldn't even realize it had occurred;
- are often leaders in the groups they belong to;
- are often in this stage more like students than they have ever been, find inspiration and education from any and all other sources;
- are not interested in gains unless it serves a deeper meaning and purpose for the greater good of humanity; and
- have invested tens or hundreds of thousands of dollars and possibly thousands of hours into their learning and unlearning.

Sage Benchmarks

- Eighteen to Twenty-Four-Plus Books/E-books/Audiobooks per Year

As mentioned in all the previous stages, reading and delving deeper into the wisdom and education of others is crucial. At this stage, some people may even have written a book or multiple books as a form of contribution to their deeper purpose. Consuming a book a fortnight or a book a week is a common part of this person's mental diet.

- Two to Four-Plus Weeks of Training Courses or Equivalent

People at this stage will devote a chunk of their year about up to a month or more in courses and possibly even to educating and teaching those courses. Courses can come in the form of spiritual retreats, business breakthroughs, or leadership skills.

- One Hundred-Plus Hours of Mood Prep/Quiet Time per Year

Their 50-to-20-minutes-a-day minimum becomes as important as any of their meals, their training sessions, or even their work. They won't see a difference between time for themselves in mood prep or meditation as it is all part of a bigger integration of their health and their purpose. To take it away would be the same as taking food or even work away from them.

Overall, these benchmarks are guidelines for development. One of the best ways to move through these stages, like with other stages, is education and coaching. Whether it be physical, nutritional, or mental, coaching is one of the fastest ways to move through any stage of development.

Over the coming chapters, I will share with you some models and insights into helping you understand yourself on an even deeper level and also helping you identify behaviors and patterns in your thinking that can help rewire the way you view yourself, others, and the world.

I will also be sharing a number of books that I highly recommend reading if you find these topics interesting. Understanding them on deeper levels allows us to understand ourselves on a deeper level. If you are curious and would like to learn more about these and yourself, then you are more than welcome to reach out to me and learn more about my programs at www.davenixon.com.au or www.bossfit.online.

An Integral Approach

Arguably one of the best philosophers and thought leaders of the 20th and 21st centuries is Ken Wilber. Ken has often been referred to as "the Einstein of consciousness studies," and his most notable work is called "integral theory."

Integral theory is a framework of human knowledge and human experience in a four-quadrant grid. This model allows us to see an integrated view of health. The model itself can be used for just about anything from political structures to psychology. We will be using it to get an integrated view of health and help expand our

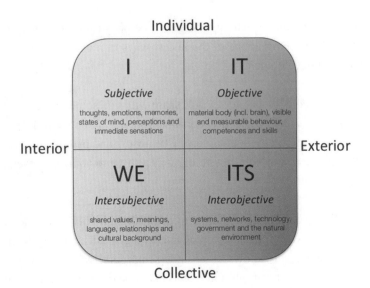

awareness of all the factors that go into maintaining a high level of HIQ.

The four domains, or "quadrants," are known as upper left, lower left, upper right, and lower right. At the top of the y-axis is the word "individual," at the bottom of the y-axis is the word "collective," to the left of the x-axis is the word "interior," otherwise known as subjective, and to the right of the x-axis is the word "exterior" or "objective."

We want to look at our health from an integral viewpoint, and this is by far the best model I have found to truly break down the different areas of health and all the implications to it. There will be quadrants we are strong in, and they will feel very familiar or even native, and then other quadrants may feel unfamiliar, undertrained, or even wrong.

Subjective Quadrant (MIND in HIQ Map)

The upper left quadrant is known as the subjective domain. This is where the individual and interior domains meet, and this domain represents all the subjective parts of our health, our thoughts, values, beliefs, as well as our emotional awareness, maturity, and intelligence. If we are physically fit but have ignored the subjective areas, then are we really healthy? Visually, on the outside, it would appear so. But, like a tall tree with shallow roots, it will come crashing down. To quote Carl Jung (who funnily enough would fall into the UL domain from a psychology point of view), "No tree, it is said, can grow to heaven unless its roots reach down to hell." To master this domain is to understand ourselves, our deep and sometimes unconscious intentions behind our actions and behaviors. This area can be one of the hardest to develop due to the fact that it is so hard to measure. That aside, this domain can be the most courageous to uncover. This is where childhood traumas and childhood patterns can be found hiding. This is the domain that can hold the answers to what we are really searching for. One of the most powerful ways to approach the subjective domain is through questions. An effective coach or someone in one of the psych fields can be invaluable in really understanding our own minds.

Often, seeing a psychologist (or someone similar) carries a stigma that the person is crazy. It's not true; I don't know anyone who wouldn't benefit from working with a trained professional in understanding themselves better. Seeing a psychologist or someone similar is no different from getting advice from a personal fitness instructor. There is no shame in getting assistance in understanding the complexities of the human mind. In the same way, there is no shame in getting some guidance in understanding the complexities of the human body.

Intersubjective (MIND in the HIQ Map)

The lower left quadrant is known as the intersubjective domain. This domain represents everything that is subjectively shared. It can reflect culture, a sense of community, mutual understanding, shared values, and relationships. From a HIQ perspective, it will reflect the people you decide to spend your time with and what their relationship brings to the table and, of course, what your relationship brings them. It will reflect the communities and culture of the workplaces you are in. It will also include the healthiness of your most intimate relationships.

Are there conversations that you are avoiding having with business partners? Spouses? Family members? Although it is possible, it is challenging to have a healthy mind and be within an "unhealthy" community. An integration of both can yield some of the most rewarding changes you may ever experience. This is truly what it means to be around like-minded people. If you are fascinated by particular things and learning or doing those things makes you feel more alive, then getting around people who have similar interests can drastically improve your life and also aid in giving you a sense of belonging, family, and contribution.

"Before you diagnose yourself with depression or low self-esteem, first make sure you are not, in fact, just surrounded by assholes." It could be Sigmund Freud who said this. Could be some lady called Debi Hope. Either way, make sure you are not one of the assholes.

Objective (MOVE in the HIQ Map)

The upper right quadrant is known as the objective domain. This domain represents everything that is objective and present in the perceived world. This is where "things out there" exist. This is also where our body exists, as well as our behaviors and skills. When we develop this area, we give ourselves freedom to express and participate in life to whatever degree we wish. Exercise isn't so much about how much you weigh or how much weight you can move; it is about how much life you can experience. When we begin training with that in mind, we liberate ourselves from the numbers on the scales and the numbers on the bar and start counting the memories.

One of the few exceptions of this is when weight classes or total weight lifted in sports are integral to a successful career. Too often we see short-term amateur athletes putting their bodies through grueling training and ending up with long-term injuries or issues that didn't outweigh the rewards of being an amateur athlete.

Developing mastery of the objective domain is developing mastery of the body. A six-week challenge cannot give you this. Nope, not even 12 weeks. It is a lifelong relationship. And, oh, what a beautiful relationship it can be.

Interobjective (MOUTH in the HIQ Map)

The lower right quadrant is known as the interobjective domain, and it represents the exterior collective systems and structures as well as the objective systemic structures of nature and humankind. For the HIQ, this is where we start to look at nutrition. We want to see whether it is a cultural fit, so that could be seen as eating locally farmed produce and also understanding that we are consuming a collection of objects from the world that are consumable. When we start to have a deeper understanding of nutrition and where our food comes from, we start to make better and better choices, not just for our mental health and our physical health but also for the environment and the world as a whole.

As you will see in the nutrition chapters, developing our nutritional HIQ is a process like anything else. We can't go from knowing very little to eating a perfect diet. And if we try, we often yo-yo and then think something is wrong with us. There isn't; you wouldn't take tenth-grade math in your second year of schooling. It takes time to learn what you need to learn to get to where you want to go, to embody the information, and be healthy nutritionally.

The Reductionist View

One of the dangers of our beloved fitness and health industry is the reductionist view that "experts" can often take when promoting their products or information. They will promote that they have the best training program or the best diet challenge. This type of reductionist view can leave us open to failures and susceptible to making the same mistakes as before due to reducing health down to a diet, an exercise regime or something else external to ourselves.

An integral view of health allows us to see how an integration of all the areas of health supports us to maintain a healthy outlook on life and have a true holistic approach to our health. We stop seeing the physical and mental as separate and see that it is an intertwined web of beauty and experience, that they are constantly cause-and-effecting upon each other. So to be healthy, as you can see, we must integrate it all.

The mental component to our health is so integral to our overall health and well-being, yet it is so often undervalued, misunderstood, or just overlooked. If there is just one thing that you take from this book, take the importance of the continual development and training of your mind, emotions, and thoughts and continue to see that understanding yourself is a forever unfolding process wrapped in beauty, fear, vulnerability, and love.

Unbecome Who You're Not

In order to get to the next level or stage of development, we have to let go of whom we think we are that got us this far. Sometimes the thing that holds us back is the very thing that got us to where we are. This is why it is so difficult to change habits or thinking patterns because at some point they served us. Otherwise we would have never of developed them. At some point in our life they yielded a positive response, so we kept doing it. Unfortunately, as we get older, our habits and thinking patterns may not work as well in all situations. For example, someone who gets angry quickly may have grown in a household that valued the ability to stand up for themselves and fight. Because of that, as they get older, the nurtured response is to get defensive even when there isn't anything to defend or they aren't even being attacked. Although as a child this helped them find safety and maybe even significance, as an adult it can destroy relationships and cause tension in everyday situations as the person is almost looking for something to defend themselves against. This is just one in a myriad of examples. Some people may even think that getting angry or anger itself is inherently bad, so they avoid it, suppress it even. Anger is an emotion just like any other. People can be quick to jump in and say they hate emotional people. Do they hate happy people? What about shameful people? What about love? When we box emotions into negative and positive, we do damage to the utility of those emotions. Anger is a very normal and very valid emotion. It points to something that possibly might put us or others in danger, and it also allows us to tap into a form of energy we don't otherwise have access to in extreme situations. Its utility is not as obvious in today's society, but human beings have been around for a long time, and you are the successor of someone who either had a choice of being killed or killing something. You can probably thank your ancestors that they allowed themselves to access their anger, otherwise you may not be here today. Now just to be clear, it is frowned upon to kill something when you're angry. Unless it's a workout.

So at some point in this person's life, they saw anger as a useful emotion to keep them safe. So later on in life, when they want to feel safe, they will do the same thing. Some people do this by serving. In today's society that seems like a nicer gesture and selfless, but if the person's intention is to get someone to like them so that they are safe, then are they truly being selfless and are they truly serving? Of course not, they are doing it for a return. They may not consciously see that in the moment; they just tell themselves they are being polite. But what they are actually doing is establishing a safe space.

All this feeds into our personal identity, which can be so damaging for us. As humans we seek to belong and to stand out all at the same time. So we figure out how we are different from everyone, and by doing so we end up associating with a demographic. So by separating we are simply only segregating. It is our identity that can really hold us back. Our identity is a belief, and we will uphold our beliefs so that our map of reality is in order and correct. But beliefs can change. They change all the time. Imagine being 40 and having the same belief you have when you were 9. Thirty-one years of experience is being overridden by a nine-year-old memory. So when you respond in the moment with that belief and overarching frame, you are responding as a less mature version of yourself. It lacks flexibility, and for that reason, takes us further away from living our potential.

Maybe we identify as a coach or a salesperson or even a mother. None of these are actually true. They are all things we do, they are not us. Maybe we identify as fat, as uncoordinated, or as weird. These are also not true. We aren't fat; we have fat. We also have fingernails; you are not a fingernail. Identifying as uncoordinated will keep you uncoordinated, and thinking that you're weird will help ensure that you do things that align with that belief so that everything is right in the world, when we all know that secretly you like being weird. So, in short, for us to become who we truly are, we must first unbecome whom we are not.

So if we are stripping away this identity? Who are we?

Have you ever noticed that there is the voice in the head and then there is the thing in your head that hears the voice in your head? Now can you see that there is something witnessing the voice in your head being heard by the part that is hearing it?

That is the witness.

The observer.

That is you.

You are the observer of the thoughts, the emotions, the world. The observer doesn't judge; it doesn't speak; it doesn't think.

It observes.

This is us.

The trouble is we often identify as the thoughts in our heads. They must be my thoughts. "If I think bad thoughts, I must be bad. If I think good thoughts, I must be good." Think good thoughts, be good. You're not your thoughts. They probably aren't even your thoughts anyway. I have spoken to countless people who tell me their limiting beliefs only to realize that they aren't even their thoughts. They were beliefs gifted to them by their caretakers, teachers, or coaches. They didn't come up with it. The self-limiting belief was passed on from generation to generation and each person owned it because they identify as the voice in their head.

Let me say this one more time; you are not your thoughts; you are not your body. You have thoughts and you have a body; that is not you. You are the silent observer. You are the witness.

By learning to identify as the witness, we start to step back and see our thoughts and see our emotions as not being what we are. It is fascinating to note that we don't see the world as it is; we see the world as we are. All our perceptual filters alter the way we see the world and contribute to the multitude of different views people have of the world. These were mostly developed in childhood and yielded a positive response for us, so we continued to develop them and over time they became familiar.

One of the other traps people fall into is identifying as their body. They see their personal worth as how healthy they appear to others, whether or not they have a six-pack, a big booty, a tan. You are not your body in the same way that when you are driving a car, you are not the car. You are inside the car, but you are not the car. The body, like the car, is a vehicle that can get you from one place to another. Your personal worth does not depend on what the car looks like, and if you look after your car, then you can usually get more kilometers out of it without having any major surgeries.

Our identity will more often get in the way of our development, and one of the most important things we can do is to really listen to how we label ourselves, even if it is only to ourselves. What does our internal dialogue sound like? "I can't do that," "I am just not like that," "I have always been this way," "They don't know what I have been through."

The idea of good and bad emotions is dangerous. Like I mentioned earlier, when we segregate emotions into good and bad emotions, we do what we can to avoid the bad ones and do what we can to gain more of the good ones. So much so we stop trying to hear and see what the so-called bad ones point out. So we shut them up by distracting ourselves, drugging ourselves, or numbing ourselves. The emotions that we call negative like anxiousness, fear, sadness, anger, and so on are all simply pointing at something important. The emotions are sending us information about our experience of the world. It is crazy to think that we just ignore that because it feels yucky. Happiness, joyfulness, confidence, and other positive emotions are also sending us information. People can take the information as "Feels yucky. Don't do that again" or "Feels amazing. Do that again." This doesn't work so well if you decide to take illegal drugs that send your body a bucketload of dopamine. It's an expensive way to lose weight.

You know there is a funny thing about anxiety or depression. They can be quite complicated, personal, and emotional topics, but it is so crucial to understand the two disorders. It is also equally important to know that for most of us, they aren't disorders. They are in order. They have become a reaction for us to particular things, people, thoughts, or events in life that we have developed over the years. Like a skill or a trade, we practiced the same order of reactions. The order works perfectly; it may just not be getting us the results we want in life. Let's shed some light on this for the moment, and let's also reaffirm that there are individual cases where anxiety and depression are clinical disorders, I am not talking about these. I am talking about the everyday hero whom we pass in the streets, who is dealing with these responses from day to day, yet was never taught how to understand them and work through them.

Think about how people talk about anxiety for a moment. The gym makes me anxious; thinking about going out gives me anxiety. Every time he rings I get anxiety. Have you heard any of these before? Or maybe similar statements? Maybe you know someone who says these types of things or maybe you fall into this category as well. Either way, I am here to break it to you that none of these things can give you anxiety. Things can't give you anything. They are just things, events, or thoughts. Anxiousness is your trained response to these things. When we blame events, things, people, or thoughts for giving us anxiety, we become the victims and look to move away from the "thing" that we think gave us the anxiety. We do this to protect ourselves; it makes so much sense. But what it really does is make us weaker, not in the way that someone is not worthy, but in the way where we never truly learn to master our minds and our emotions. Anxiousness is an emotion that we have within us. It is our meaning structures and thoughts about states and states about thoughts that embeds this. Before we know it, our order of response to something is anxiousness, and we do it so damn well that it happens almost automatically.

Things don't give you anxiety; they can't. They are things. We have simply trained ourselves to respond that way.

When we realize this, we realize we can, over time, train ourselves to respond in a different manner—if we want to. Anxiousness also has a very valid and useful purpose; it points to our potential. We don't get anxious about things that can't happen. And often it is the things we need to develop that we get anxious about. That means that when anxiousness arises in us, it is often pointing at the very thing that if we developed, would move us closer to our potential. Anxiousness doesn't mean move away from, it often means move toward it. This also explains why nervousness and anxiousness have a similar sensation to excitement. The sensation is simply the body's response, whether we call it excitement or anxiousness is really up to us.

When we suppress some emotions, we learn to suppress all emotions. Emotions are normal and to be understood, not ignored. We cannot become emotionally intelligent if we continue to ignore, shun, or shame away our emotions. One of the key things to mastering our minds is mastering our understanding of what our emotions are pointing toward and accepting the wide spectrum of emotions. Intelligence comes from the Latin word *intelligere*, which means "to understand." People can often get confused with emotional intelligence and think that it means to understand and read other people. Although this may be a factor in emotional intelligence; it is shallow in its description. Emotional intelligence is to understand self, from there we can start to truly understand others. We can only meet someone as deep as we have met ourselves. We cannot understand someone else's subjective experience, if we have suppressed our emotions and allowed our thoughts to control us. We must first seek to understand self, and along that journey we will start to truly understand those around us.

So to become who we truly are and lean into our potential we must develop emotional intelligence of self and understand our four personal powers that are within our control: speech, behavior, thoughts, and emotions.

Our Personality

There are a number of different types of personality tests and ways to break down people's personality traits. A common problem with personality types is that we view them as static: this is the personality of someone and that's just who they are. But we aren't a personality; we don't even have a personality. We do personality.

Our personality is a mask made up of behavioral traits and thoughts that we have developed to deal with reality. It is not right; it is not wrong, and it just is. We developed characteristics that allowed us to feel safe and to get our needs met when we were young. What this often means is that a lot of us are walking around behaving and thinking in a way that served us when we were young but may not serve us so well as an adult. What this also means is that each and every one of us experiences reality differently through our subjective experience, which is based off many different perceptual filters and thinking patterns that were mostly developed in childhood and adolescence.

So what does this all mean for us? Well, the best model I have found to understand personality and also understand how our personality can get in the way of our potential is the Enneagram.

The Enneagram is both a horizontal and vertical model of viewing the differing types of personalities. What this means is that it shows the different types of personalities with none better or worse than others, even playing a field (horizontal, and then shows the nine levels of healthiness for each type and how they may borrow qualities and characteristics from other types depending on their level of healthiness and personal development. This is the vertical part of the Enneagram as a developmental model.

The Enneagram shows us a path of development for our type. It speaks about personality as something we do, not something we are. It is more of a psychospiritual model than a personality indicator. The Enneagram breaks down personality into nine main types. Rather than being one type, we have the capabilities of all the nine types within us. I use the three main typologies that someone would lean into as part of their developmental work to help understand themselves better.

Don Riso and Russ Hudson have been two of the modern pioneers and teachers of the Enneagram and have developed a questionnaire you can complete for a small fee to get scores back on which types you would lean into the most. There are free tests that can give a rough estimate and, over time, the better you can understand the behaviors and intentions behind all types, you may not need the test at all. After all, the state you are in will also impact the results. The test will also give you a snapshot of yourself, even though the Enneagram and I preach that you are a dynamic process that is unfolding. That said, our results won't change drastically when tests are taken again a year or more down the track. They are likely to vary slightly in results, but the core of our results will stay the same due to our typology being ingrained from such a young age.

The test I recommend to take is called the RHETI test and can be found at https://www.enneagraminstitute.com/rheti.

Now you can use any personality test to get a greater grasp of your personality and underlying intentions behind your actions, I highly recommend the Enneagram for the reasons stated as well as the large amount of information available on it to help deepen your understanding of the model and yourself.

All my personal clients will have done the test at some point, and it is something that I will coach to a fair bit. We will be using it as the standard in this book for understanding ourselves from a personality standpoint.

One thing that is important to remember with the Enneagram is that we have all the types within us. It is almost like we all have the same ingredients but differing amounts of those ingredients, which aids in giving us our uniqueness. From our youth, we have overdeveloped and valued some behavioral traits and underdeveloped and disregarded others. What this means is that we developed a lot of our personality, while we were in pursuit of things such as safety, love, connection, or acceptance. If we act in a particular way, we receive that particular thing be it safety or significance, and so we learn to continue to behave in that way, even as an adult, where it doesn't always work in the big wide world. When we were younger, we just went about getting these things from our caretakers and the world in particular ways. Then we became good at it, and it became ingrained in us and became what we call our personality. Hence why we do personality, rather than have one.

The Personality Types

There are number of books on the Enneagram that further break down the typology and the model as a whole. The goal of sharing it with you in brief here is to give you an overview of the types and some snippets about them. As mentioned before, I highly recommend taking the RHETI test, and if you are keen on reading more, then starting with *The Wisdom of the Enneagram* by Riso and Hudson, which is one of my favorites.

Once again, the importance of understanding these types is to first learn more about ourselves and then use our knowledge to understand others better. I remember hearing once that there are no difficult people, just hurt people. When we can understand where we come from and how our pain has manifested in our behaviors over years to protect us and seek out things like acceptance, then we can understand that others are simply doing the same thing, just in their own way.

There are nine basic types of the Enneagram. Each typology has its unique characteristics that are more native and familiar to that type. Each type also has a type that will gain access to when that person is under stress (disintegration) as well as another type, which will gain access when that same person is feeling secure (integration). We call these two types a path of integration or path of disintegration. We have access to each of these types' characteristics based on either being stress or secure.

For example, a type 8 (the Challenger) when healthy will take on some qualities of the type 2 (the Helper). The eight may look similar to a type 2 and can be easily misidentified as a type 2, but at their core, they are still very much a type 8. Think of it like a milkshake. Type 8 is the milkshake, and type 2 is the strawberry flavoring. It changes the taste but doesn't change the fact that it is still a milkshake.

Type 1
The Reformer or Perfectionist

Characteristics: rational, idealistic, principled, determined, self-controlled, and perfectionistic.

The reformer has a strong sense of morals and right and wrong. Reformers can often be the most judgmental of all the types although this is often toward themselves. When healthy, the type 1 is known to be a social reformer. They will be community leaders and pursue what is morally right and support what will be for the greater good. They are ethical, highly rational, and disciplined. They can be extraordinarily wise and have a noble vision and purpose.

An average reformer will take it upon themselves to try and make everything right. Of course, it can be right only in their eyes, and they can get quite upset with those who don't uphold the same amount of personal or social integrity. They will promote causes and work toward the way things "should" be. Of course, they are projecting their own values and way of living upon a greater community or society and compare what they are doing right and what others are doing wrong and must be fixed. They can start to experience bouts of depression and become workaholics.

An unhealthy reformer will become unreasonable and angry with the world but mostly with themselves. They will feel they are at fault or imperfect and go about trying to fix the systems of the world to make up for their sense of inadequacy. Everyone else is lazy or corrupt and most importantly wrong. They are extremely self-righteous, critical, and judgmental.

Path of integration: when secure and safe, the reformer will take on the qualities of the enthusiast and become lighthearted, relaxed, social, and playful.

Path of disintegration: when under stress, the reformer will take on traits of the individualist and become romantic about their own negative feelings and will often isolate themselves.

Type 2
The Helper

Characteristics: caring, interpersonal, demonstrative, generous, people pleasing, coercive, and possessive

The helper is a compassionate, empathetic, and caring type. At their healthiest they are unselfish and will freely give unconditional love with no expectation of return. They are also truly humble and charitable. They have unconditional self-worth and don't rely on external validation to feel good about themselves.

An average helper is often overly caring and overly responsible. They will find their self-worth in being constantly helpful and useful, but where they struggle is when they don't check with those they think they're helping. Often they will mind read and attempt to be helpful when in reality they aren't being helpful at all.

At the unhealthy range, the helper can become possessive, under responsible, and even develop stalker traits whether that be on social media or in person. At this stage they can even seek out people who are in desperate long-term need of help so that they are able to continually feed their desire for being needed by someone externally to fulfil their self-worth.

Path of integration: When healthy, the helper takes on the qualities of the individualist and starts to get more in touch with their own feelings and become emotionally honest and aware of their spectrum of feelings.

Path of disintegration: when under stress the helper will take on the traits of the challenger and regress to outbursts of anger and blame. They can become dominating in pursuit of what they want, which is usually around the need to be noticed as helpful or useful to others.

Type 3
The Achiever

Characteristics: success oriented, pragmatic, adaptive, excelling, driven, manipulative, and image conscious

The achiever is a noble and hardworking type who, when they allow themselves to be vulnerable, become great leaders and inspiring role models. They have an increasing desire to achieve for the greater good and larger community/world. These types can be high spirited, highly confident, popular, and attractive. At their best they are humble and honorable.

An average achiever is often concerned about how they are showing up in the world in the eyes of others and can often stretch the truth or even put on an act to hide the real them in order to be perceived to be more successful than they actually are. At their core, they are scared of being found out or having flaws. They can become manipulative in order to get what they want, tricking both themselves and the other people into thinking that it is the best for everyone. At this level, their charm turns into coercion.

An unhealthy achiever is desperate to continue to show the world that they are indeed a superior person and will go to extremes in an attempt to prove this. They may create false appointments or make up lies to make them appear busier and more important than they actually are. Pathological liars, they can become more devious and dishonest so that their faults and misconduct will remain a secret.

Path of integration: When healthy, the achiever takes on the qualities of the loyalist and begins to trust themselves and others. They move from a competitive frame of mind to a cooperative frame of mind.

Path of disintegration: When unhealthy and under stress, achievers can burn out and take on the average qualities of the peacemaker. They become vague and uninterested in their goals and life. Ultimately, they become less responsible for themselves and apathetic.

Type 4
The Individualist

Characteristics: sensitive, withdrawn, profoundly creative, expressive, dramatic, self-absorbed, and temperamental

The individualist is the romantic, artistic, and expressive type. At their healthiest, they are loving, they are self-expressive, and they have a profound ability to turn all experiences into something valuable. They are deeply reflective and emotionally strong.

An average individualist can become a little more self-absorbed and do what they can to prolong their feelings. They may take time out away from people and society to work through their feelings more before remerging. Everything can become an overindulgence in passion, emotion, or romance. They can also become more sensitive and make others walk on eggshells around them.

An unhealthy type 4 becomes isolated, and they will reject anything and anyone who doesn't uphold their idea of their own self-image. They can be drunk on their inner world and neglect how their actions may be impacting people around them. Unhealthy individualists can often live in the past and bring a lot of the past to the present moment. They can even go as far as being completely unable to take care of themselves in an attempt to elicit care for someone else, all the while complaining that they are not being taken care of adequately.

Path of integration: a healthy individualist will take on the qualities of a reformer and start to realize that rules also apply to them. They will start to make decisions objectively rather than subjectively; they become more self-disciplined rather than self-indulgent.

Path of disintegration: When unhealthy, the individualist will take on the traits of the average helper. They people please, call attention to the good things they have done for their loved ones, and look for compliments of worthiness in return.

Type 5
The Investigator

Characteristics: intense, cerebral, visionaries, perceptive, innovative, secretive, detached, and isolated

The investigator is the most cerebral of all the types. They love learning and will often become experts in their field due to their near obsessive personal interest in how things work. They are often extremely detailed and precise. They feel emotionally connected to the world as a whole and can become legendary visionaries.

The average investigator can develop a less than healthy obsession with their craft, oftentimes forgetting the actual time and also partially isolating themselves. Although that will rarely be a conscious behavior, they may be struggling with some area in their life, and they will avoid dealing with it by delving deeper into what makes them deeply interested, thus turning away from life and prolonging their issues. They remain extremely studious and often specialize in something. This can also encourage them to continue to study and never end up fulfilling their ideas in the real world.

An unhealthy investigator will be heavily introverted and retreat into their ideas in their mind as a way of escaping reality. They can become rather strange and reclusive and even mentally unstable. This is literally the archetype of the mad scientist. They can experience grave depression and fall prey to nihilism.

Path of integration: A healthy investigator will take on the qualities of a challenger and become outwardly expressive, helpful, and assertive. They will give life to their ideas and become confident leaders and will use their expertise and insight compassionately for the greater good.

Path of disintegration: an unhealthy investigator will take on the traits of the average type 7 and become scattered and ungrounded. They may continually get excited about their ideas yet never finish any of them while jumping from project to project. They stop thinking clearly and act out of impulse.

Type 6
The Loyalist

Characteristics: committed, security-oriented, engaging, supportive, responsible, anxious, and suspicious

The healthy loyalist can be cooperative, trusting, and self-confident. They are great supporters, planners, and organizers. Highly reliable and trustworthy, they are hardworking, loyal, and courageous. At their best, they can act even when faced with their doubts and fears.

An average loyalist can become cautious and suspicious of others. They lack trust in themselves and will seek something external to find their stability and support. They will often seek approval or advice from outside sources that they deem to be stable and as holding authority. They can even become suspicious of the very people they seek stability from. This is a reflection of what is going on for them on the inside as they struggle to trust themselves. The average six is the most anxious of all the types and will constantly try to plan and organize the world around them in order to alleviate this anxiety.

An unhealthy loyalist allows stress to become a way of life and get infatuated with meeting what they perceive to be important commitments and responsibilities even if it is detrimental to their long-term health and relationships. They may develop fears of abonnement and insufficiency, which will cause them to distance themselves further from others in order to avoid getting hurt, which, inadvertently, deepens their hurt. They can become paranoid as a form of protection against others and the world out there.

Path of integration: when secure and safe, loyalists become warm and self-confident. They don't need to trust others because they trust themselves. This doesn't mean they won't trust others but rather they will lean into their personal authority more and trust themselves to trust others.

Path of disintegration: when stressed and unhealthy, loyalists take on the average traits of the achiever. They can reassure everyone that they are fine while really fighting a battle on the inside. Although a lot of their battles may come from indecisiveness and not knowing whom and when to trust; ultimately, they won't trust themselves. They will keep a hard exterior and refuse help even when they need it the most.

Type 7
The Enthusiast

Characteristics: busy, joyful, fun loving, positive, spontaneous, versatile, hyperactive, distractible, and scattered

Extremely optimistic and social, the enthusiast loves to talk about ideas, brainstorm, and look at the bright side of life. At their healthiest, enthusiasts are measured, energetic, grounded, and level-headed. They have an immense ability to see good and bad and to remain hopeful during tough times.

An average enthusiast can become scattered, experience continual fear of missing out (FOMO) and fall into the trap of positivism. They can become excessive in their desire to constantly want to experience new experiences and find lighthearted ways to distract them from responsibilities and emotional maturity. Although versatile and spontaneous, this can lead to sporadic bursts of effort and constant daydreaming about the future. They are never quite there as they are constantly thinking of the next appointment, weekend, or job offer.

An unhealthy enthusiast can become manic and unreasonable in their pursuits of the next best thing. Their constant desire for external stimulus can leave them feeling numb and unable to connect to themselves, especially in the present moment. If you scratch a 7, you get a 6. What this means is that type 7s can be just as anxious as the 6s; however, instead of trying to organize everything in order to keep their anxiety at bay, they constantly distract themselves with pleasures, constant chatter, and even denial of reality in favor of unjustified positivism.

Path of integration: when healthy, the enthusiast will take on the qualities of the investigator. They will become measured and think clearly before acting. They are able to channel their energy toward a worthy goal or pursuit with a laser focus.

Path of disintegration: when under stress, the enthusiast will revert to the traits of an average reformer. They can grow increasingly anxious and frustrated with themselves about the amount of work or "things to do" that can pile up and become extremely critical of self and rude to others in an attempt to get their life in order. If they are not careful, this will only be temporary until they escape or distract themselves again, only to feel worse about not being able to see something through.

Type 8
The Challenger or the Boss

Characteristics: powerful, dominating, self-confident, strong, natural leaders, decisive, potentially violent, and confrontational

The challenger can be the most supportive, compassionate, and the natural leaders among all the types. When healthy, they can be forthright yet empathetic and use their strength and will for the greater good of society and the planet. Best said by Riso and Hudson to be truly fearless, challengers are willing to put themselves in jeopardy to achieve a vision: possibly heroic and historically great.

An average 8 can be to the point and lack empathy and sympathy for others. They can value hard work over health and can often be disconnected to their body and experience burn out. They can become angry and constantly blame others for the mistakes of the world around them. They have a constant desire to be independent and as tough as possible although this is mostly a front. It is their way or the highway as they protect themselves by ignoring emotions that may appear to make them weak, which, inadvertently, is a weakness

An unhealthy 8 is most likely to be violent and can express anger easily. They despise any attempt to be controlled even if it is by the law and can often become renegades, con artists, and outlaws. This can lead them to become ruthless and be feared, which both deepens their desire to protect themselves and to appear strong or fearful in the eyes of others. They see everything as a challenge and a fight or battle, one they must win, no matter what.

Path of integration: a healthy challenger takes on the qualities of the helper and develops the ability to use their energy, strength, and leadership skills to help develop those in their community, society, or on a global level. They are formidable for a great cause and are brave leaders.

Path of disintegration: under stress 8s can take on the traits of an average investigator. When they feel overwhelmed, they can become reclusive and introverted, often disappearing to regather information, plans, and strategies to feel confident enough to move forward again. This can also cause them to feel even more rejected by those around them and even the world.

Type 9
The Peacemaker

Characteristics: easygoing, self-effacing, receptive, reassuring, agreeable, daydreaming, and complacent

A healthy peacemaker is confident and cooperative while also driven and self-assured. They are genuinely kind people and have a sense of ease about them but can also be to the point without appearing rude. When they form healthy relationships with themselves and continue to keep their inner peace, they are able to form honest and deep personal relationships with other people. They can become exuberant and full of life.

An average peacemaker will often do what they can to keep the peace within. They will attempt to do this by keeping the peace outside. They may fall into the trap that their stability and peace is based on external things or circumstances, which is still very much a childhood pattern of pleasing the parents or completely zoning out in order to be at peace. They may zone out via video games, movie binges, or even daydreaming. They sometimes confuse this escapist mentality with being easy going, when in reality it is much harder for everyone else in the long term. They may also escape by having busy routines and being emotionally disconnected with their day-to-day activities while waiting for something to change.

An unhealthy peacemaker can often have a deep-down rage that they are attempting to keep under control. They learn to suppress their emotions because if it were to boil over, then everything would come crashing down and, of course, there would be no peace. They can become angry or extremely upset with anyone who tries to point out their stress level or unhealthy behaviors and can even fall into the trap of blaming the person who is attempting to help them. In this space, they can become less responsible and neglectful to those who may rely on them.

Path of integration: a healthy peacemaker takes on the qualities of a healthy achiever. They lean into their self-confidence and ability to be task orientated and make things happen and show up in the world.

Path of disintegration: a peacemaker under stress can take on the average traits of the loyalist and become untrusting and anxious. They may continue to blame others in a way to deal with their struggles. Paradoxically, they also become more needful of others in this space.

Levels of Healthiness

The vertical development component of the Enneagram is the levels of healthiness. Healthiness can also be explained as levels of integration. The term "integration" refers to how well this person has integrated all of their personality, shadows, and other areas of their psyche that they may have once rejected. When we integrate all the parts of us we don't like, we move into acceptance and can truly start to focus on becoming a better individual not only for ourselves but also for our community. When we are at war with ourselves, we are at war with others.

There are nine levels of healthiness. Levels 1, 2, and 3 are the healthiest and reflect what those types are like when they are less constricted by their egoic structures and more present and closer to their true essence. People at this level have often done a hell of a lot of self-work. Unfortunately, there isn't a short cut to being able to overcome and eliminate a lot of the patterns developed when we were young, besides working through them. It takes time. It can be really hard and really painful. But it won't be more painful than taking all our baggage with us throughout our life. A lot of the patterns that were handed to us when we were younger were also traits of our parents. We have the opportunity through self-work or personal development to end the cycle of limiting beliefs and codependent relationships. We have the opportunity to free the next generation from as much unnecessary suffering as possible through relieving ourselves from it. There is no short cut. There is no finish line. There is no magic pill. There is just the truth that is no longer influenced by your "truth."

Levels 4, 5, and 6 show the traits of each type when they are at an average level of healthiness. This is where most people whom you come into contact with each day will sit. Levels 4 and 5 are the most average whereas level 6 can either be a disintegration and defragmentation of ourselves and psyches before dropping into unhealthy levels or it can be a higher level for those of us recovering from being in unhealthy levels.

We all have a bandwidth that shows where we would reach in our healthiest state compared to the lower levels we have access to when under a lot of stress. Later on in the book, I use this same type of indication when it comes to nutrition. Each day brings new adventures and challenges, and we have our own difficulties and perceptions of reality to work through. Because of the dynamic nature of life, we also have a dynamic nature toward it. You may have peak state access to a higher level such as a 2 or

3 and then when under a lot of stress, drop down into a 5. This is normal; the work is in continually being able to be aware of ourselves and how we choose to show up and respond to each moment.

Levels 7, 8, and 9 are the unhealthy levels. These levels are often dangerous for those who are in it and possibly even those close to the person who is experiencing these levels. In these levels we are at the mercy of our egoic structures and have fallen into despair, depression, and possibly self-destruction. In these levels, it is advisable to seek professional help from psychologists or therapists. There is no shame in doing so. We all need help from time to time, and sometimes seeing someone can be the bravest thing we can do. Not just for us, but also our loved ones.

For further reading on the levels of healthiness please refer to the books mentioned in the next chapter.

Finding Your Type

As mentioned earlier, we don't have a personality; we do a personality. The beautiful thing about the Enneagram is that it expresses nine different types, which we all have access to. So we aren't any one type. We are made up of all the types. We just strong in and familiar toward a couple of them. This means that there are some types that we do really well and are familiar with, and other types that we may struggle to relate to. The reason why we would say "do really well" is for the most part because our personality is something that we do, not something we have.

You may have related to a couple of the types when reading through them. People who are trained in using the Enneagram are often able to pick types just from conversations and observing behaviors. The idea is to steer away from trying to type people as it can become more harmful than helpful. What I recommend is form an idea of what type you may think someone is and then encourage them to do the test and compare that with your initial thoughts.

Once again you can use any personality indicator that you like. If you wish to go further down the Enneagram path then I recommend first doing the test at the following website: https://www.enneagraminstitute.com/rheti. It will take 40 minutes, cost about $12, and also give you a 30-page report of your results.

If you still are interested in learning more, once that is complete then any books by Don Riso and Russ Hudson is a great place to start. My three recommendations are

- *The Wisdom of the Enneagram*
- *Personality Types*
- *Understanding the Enneagram*

Above everything, this will give you a greater level of insight into yourself and how you may respond to the world under stress and when feeling secure and also give you recommendations for a path of development. It can point to childhood patterns that would have likely been developed from common patterns that happen in our lives and how to mature through the levels of healthiness to move toward your ultimate potential and essence.

It is extremely challenging to truly reach our potential without truly knowing ourselves. I highly encourage you to invest the time and energy into learning more about yourself. It is one of the most selfless things you can do.

Mindful Mindset

I have honestly done my best to avoid using the word "mindful" throughout this book. You could even say that I have been . . . mindful of it.

At the moment, mindfulness is in fashion. From hashtags and brands to mindfulness classes, and of course, books—it is everywhere. The interesting thing about mindfulness isn't the desired outcome that most people want to gain from it, or even what a lot of people may teach when talking about it. The issue comes with the fact that in today's busy world and with all the demands that life has for us, the last thing we need is a full mind.

It is not a full mind that we seek. It is an empty one. One void of stuff, things, worries, concerns, limiting beliefs, positivism, to-do lists—an empty mind. We don't even have to create one. Because that would be filling the mind with the empty one.

We already have one. The empty mind is the part of the mind that observes all the thoughts, beliefs, emotions, judgments, everything. Too often we identify as the thoughts and not the parts of the mind that observe the thoughts, or one step further, the part of the mind that observes the observation of the thoughts.

Stop and think for just a moment. There is a voice thinking, then there is something hearing that voice. And you are observing both. That is you observing. That is the empty mind. It doesn't judge, it doesn't want, it just observes. In this space we can slow down our mind, step back, and take control. We get to choose what we feel is important and useful for us. It allows us to have wisdom we didn't realize we had access to. It helps us to gain insight we otherwise would have pursued in other people.

Our other mind is already full. That's one of the problems. It is our ability to step into our empty mind and move into our personal wisdom and true self that allows us to move closer to our potential.

Maybe to some this might sound crazy. If it doesn't already, I am sure at some point it will make sense. Let's call that a peak-state experience. From there, with practice and self-work, we can continue to move into that space more and more, delving deeper into our self and the things that we are holding on to that are holding us back.

The goal is to not fill our mind; the aim is to empty it, not to slow down our thoughts, but to stop identifying as them, to observe them. This allows us to question our beliefs, to test what is actually true. To see what is serving us and to see what parts of us no longer serve us and to learn to let them go. This can help us free our mind and bring us back to the present.

The other interesting paradox is the talk around mind-set. For the most part, we don't want to set our mind. True power comes with the flexibility and adaptability of our mind, not the rigidity of it. People may even argue that you could set it to positive. Not a bad idea really; unfortunately, this is an immature way to view reality. "Positive" is simply a judgment, and it is often a static judgment. What initially seems positive may turn to be negative and vice versa.

It is our ability to realize that things just are what they are, and we use our map of reality to understand them. This is called subjective experience, which is different although it may be similar to someone else's subjective experience of the very same thing.

The point of this is to remind you that you have an opportunity in every single moment to show up as you are today, to not be set to old frames and beliefs that once served you and now have become your default response. You don't need to work hard to find the secret to mindfulness and mind-set. The truth is your mind is already empty, and your mind can be entirely adaptable to the present moment and allow you to respond in a way that serves the moment.

There is a big difference between responding in a way that serves the current moment and responding in a way that serves old beliefs and reactions. The beauty is that you get to choose.

I challenge you to swap your mindful mind-set for an empty and fluid mind that is not governed by what is required in the moment, which will allow you to experience life the most and set you up for your future emotionally, mentally, and physically.

Thinking Patterns

A group of perceptual filters we have that help us filter and make sense of reality is called Metaprograms. "Metaprograms" is really just a fancy way of saying thinking patterns. They are patterns in the way that we personally think.

Overall there are currently 60 thinking patterns that we have that help us filter reality. Out of those 60 we have about 7 (plus or minus 2) drivers that we have developed so well that we couldn't possibly comprehend a different viewpoint. These driver patterns become so ingrained in our thinking that they become the lens we view reality through. It can become extremely hard, although not impossible to identify our drivers without someone pointing them out for us. Even then, if we aren't ready to see them, we will likely reject them.

Thinking patterns can be in the form of a scale, continuum, or binary. You don't have to be just one side of the pattern, and it can be contextual. You may find it easy to be on one side of the pattern in one setting in your life and then be on the other side in another area of your life.

Understanding these patterns can allow us to step back and look at how we are currently perceiving reality. In doing so, we can start to choose how we make meaning of it. We can start to choose what we are actually paying attention to. We can start to see what we may be missing. The beauty of this is that it allows us to expand our awareness. Our potential comes from increasing our awareness, which can be considered to deepen our perspectives. To lean into our potential, we can lean into the programs and patterns we are familiar with. This is how we deepen our perspectives. First we must recognize how we are viewing reality and second we have to ask ourselves what we are missing? What would it look like from a different perspective? If I were to take a different stand on this situation, what would I see?

I am going to share the 15 most common patterns and what I think are the most important thinking patterns when it comes to our health and wellness. Now it could be argued that all patterns are important and of course they are; I am simply offering the 15 that I see the most in the gym and in coaching, which have either been at the root of their problem or have helped them make a breakthrough.

A couple of things to note when it comes to these thinking patterns is that they often work in clusters. What this means is that our opinion of something is usually a result of a cluster of programs coming together to help form that thought or position. This is important to know when looking at ourselves and finding what may be at the root of our own problems. I have two offers for you in this chapter on thinking patterns. One is to really attempt to lean into any of the programs and try out either both sides or all the positions on offer. If you struggle to lean into something that is being offered and find it extremely easy to lean into the other side, then you might find that is a driver for you.

When we find our drivers, we may even want to keep them because we think they are right. This is why they are drivers. As you will see through the next 15 patterns, there is no good or bad. It is all contextual. Patience is great when wanting to get results in the gym and remembering to play the long game. Patience may not be so great when your son is choking, and you are stuck in traffic on the way to the hospital.

These programs are not something we are or something we have; they are something we do, something that we have trained ourselves to do really well. This also means that if we want to truly develop our potential in and out of the gym, it heavily lies in our ability to lean into each side of the programs and patterns to develop and broaden our awareness. Understanding these patterns when it comes to ourselves, our environment, and our training can be pivotal in developing our mental fortitude to work through anything in life we want to. Remember, no good and bad. Just contextual.

My second offer is to learn more about the programs. If you want to learn more, then the book you want to get your hands on is *Figuring Out People* by Michael Hall. This is an extension of both his and The Coaching Rooms teachings. You can learn more about The Coaching Room at www.thecoachingroom.com.au.

Fifteen Thinking Patterns

These thinking patterns are in no particular order, and you may also find that you don't really lean into one or the other, but you lean into both sides of the pattern. That's okay, it just means it isn't a driver for you. The real key here isn't necessarily being or doing either side of the pattern. It is the ability to step back and be able to choose how you want to view each and every event and situation. That power of choice is power in itself.

1. Counting Pattern
Counting or Discounting
We are going to start with one that I see as a driver all too often. Although this state is called information staging, which is

accurate, it is easier to describe it as how we see ourselves. We can discount information in the same way that we foreground and background people in a movie. The actors who are foregrounded are the main focus, and the people in the background are not. In short, they are not the main actors. They are not important, which in turn, means the actors in the foreground are important. People often do this with themselves, backgrounding themselves and their achievements and putting other people and their achievements in the foreground. Discounting can be a motivational strategy; it can be a way to not stand out or it can also be a protective mechanism. Either way, we discount ourselves in the face of someone else. When this becomes a driver, the so-called imposter syndrome kicks in, and you may feel you are punching above your weight in your relationship or nothing you do is ever good enough. You may struggle to take a compliment and deflect the compliment each time.

On the other hand, are those of us who acknowledge our strengths in a healthy way without discounting the parts of us that are developing. We acknowledge the effort we are putting in to improving without the need or desire to play it down. When we go too far into counting, we become boastful and egotistic. We might inflate our achievements in order to feel important and want to tell other people about it. This may come from a sense of not feeling important unless I am achieving and, of course, unless you know about my achieving. This bravado is fake and a mask for real confidence.

Conclusion: At its core, counting and discounting are just ways in which we stage information. What do we foreground (about ourselves, others, and information) and what do we background?

Practice: one of the main areas I see here that can be improved on is the discounting. It is really hard to lean into your potential, lead a family home, and bring up healthy kids when we constantly discount ourselves. Bring awareness to the small wins that you have. They may be more significant than you initially think. By leaning into counting the little things you do, you can really help build a strong sense of self-confidence and assurance that you may have once lost. If you only acknowledge your achievements when you finally arrive, you may be bitterly disappointed at the end, because we never arrive. That's not the point of life. The point of life is to live it, in each step.

2. Scale Pattern
Global or Detailed

This particular thinking pattern is great to get a handle on when it comes to learning how we and others communicate and see information. Some people prefer to talk about the big picture whereas others can almost get lost in the details.

People who scale information globally tend to be visionaries and can set lofty dreams without giving too much consideration to the details. "We will figure that out as we go." But they never do, because they are often about thinking the big picture and never get around to dealing with the small steps and the detail required to get there. People who scale globally will often speak globally too. Of course this is contextual, and sometimes people who are global in social settings can be detailed in personal settings and vice versa. Remember, there is no right or wrong; this is simply just a way to filter information.

People who are detailed are often in careers that support detail such as accounting or science and technology, and you would hope that your doctor is detailed when looking after your health, even if you ask for an "overview." Detailed individuals can often get caught up in the details and spreadsheets and never really have a long-term view or vision or lack big thinking. They can sometimes err on the side of being averse to risk. This can be due to the amount of data or information that shows a large percentage of risk in attempting a lot of goals. Sometimes all they will see is the tree; they won't be able to see the forest.

Conclusion: Being either global or detailed has its benefits, but where the real benefits lies is in having the ability to lean into both. Thinking macro (global) and acting micro (detail) allows us to set big-time goals and be precise in the steps that we need to take to get there. Where this can really become an issue is when we talk globally about our downfalls or about a bad day. Global communication is also known as inductive communication. What this means is that when we talk globally, especially about "bad" things that happen, we can turn something that happened once or twice into something that is permeant, pervasive, and personal. Running late for work, being cut off in traffic, and spilling your first coffee can make a global person think that it is a bad day. Even a detailed person can fall into that trap. However, sitting back and looking at the fact that running late is a normal thing and can have many factors that are out of your control involved, such as being cut off in traffic, but you're safe, and the person didn't mean it only leaves you with spilling your coffee, which didn't go on anyone and was easy to clean up. In doing so, you may have even spoken to the cute waiter whom you wouldn't have otherwise spoken to. So be very careful with trancing yourself into a negative state with global language. Pay attention to the details, it will get you out of a shitty state. Unless of course, you want to be there.

Practice: if you find that you lean into global communication, bringing awareness to vague answers or vague questions is a simple first step followed by taking the time to reword your response or question to be more precise and clearer. If you find yourself leaning more into details then learning to pay attention to the big picture, so that you know where you are going helps. Getting lost in the details means that you were so focused on the details, you literally lost sight of where you were headed. This is important in life, business, relationships, and also each day.

3. Attention Pattern Internal or External

This pattern is speaking to our point of reference or focus. Do we mainly focus on ourselves or do we focus on other people or things. Someone who does internal reference well will often go into their own world experiences and senses when relating to someone. They may even come across as selfish or self-centered, when in reality, they are just really good at internal reference. "How will this impact me?" I have a similar story to that. It was really bad timing that she went on holiday (probably not for her buddy). People who internally reference well will habitually look from their point of view first and may even completely neglect to try and understand someone else's.

Someone who leans into external reference well will have meaning such as "If everyone else is comfortable, then I am comfortable." When it comes to the gym, someone who externally references really well may not want to let the coach down and be completely disconnected from how their body is feeling. They don't want to be perceived as a quitter in someone else's eyes. Remember this is all contextual, and intent is also crucial to understand. Someone may run an external referent pattern in the gym but run an internal pattern in a relationship.

Conclusion: the real benefit is in being able to lean into both internal and external referencing. This simply means that we are able to understand whether we are owning what we feel, what we think, and are able to have the ability to inquire into the other person. This can be very beneficial when we are pursuing a new training or nutrition plan, and we can understand both what we think, feel, and want and what our significant other or even kids think, feel, and want. We are in a better position to see the whole picture rather than being out of touch with what is either important to us or them.

Practice: Giving yourself some space in a conversation or situation to ask, "Do I know what I want in this situation," or, on the flip side, "Do I know what they want in this situation" can allow you to find out what you really lean into and where you may benefit from asking more questions and gathering more data.

4. Authority Pattern
Internal authority

Internal and external authority (not to be confused with attention/ reference) is, in short, our ability to make decisions by ourselves or hand over our authority to someone else. When we do internal authority well we can really lean into our own power and trust ourselves to make a decision that will be best for us and best for our community/family. Another way to look at our personal authority is to think about it as permission. Do we look for permission externally or do we look internally for permission. This could be permission to change careers, be the person you truly want to be, or even go to the toilet. People who do internal authority well give themselves permission and hold their opinion of themselves, their worth, and their judgments in higher regard than others. This doesn't mean that they won't respect other people's points of view, and when going to an extreme, they can be completely ignore other people, and it can become damaging.

Alternatively, someone who does external authority really well will often ask other people for input and what they think they should do. When it comes to health and fitness, they will ask what programs they should do, what they should eat, if they should rest, or what weights they should do in the gym. Sometimes this is information gathering; other times it is external authority.

Conclusion: when it comes to internal and external authority, we want to be able to learn to lean into both and know when to do both. When it comes to our own health and our own well-being, making decisions and backing ourselves is the way to develop our internal authority and also to take our power back from constantly being told what to do. From a fitness standpoint, it is truly giving yourself permission to be fallible and still take what's yours, to go after what you truly want. The permission frame can sometimes sound a bit cliché, but if we don't give ourselves permission, we seek it in others. When we do that, we never play the main character in the movie that is our life.

Practice: pay attention to the conversations that you have and how often you may seek validation, permission, or approval from an external source. See how often you hand over your power, and whether someone else is making a decision that directly impacts you. Trust yourself to make decisions and that everything will be okay. It may feel strange in the beginning, but over time this will help you build confidence in yourself to do what needs to be done.

A lot of this patterning was developed in childhood and always asking for permission from authority figures. If we aren't aware of this, in our adult life, we will still seek permission from figures whom we put in that space. For those who find it challenging to hand power over, the practice would be to learn to let go. This can be one of the best practices for those who run a strong internal authority program as their need to control is often controlling them. Handing over some of that authority in small steps allows for balance in relationships and health.

5. Self-Esteem Pattern
Conditional or Unconditional

Our self-esteem is simply another way to describe our personal value. So what we want to define is whether or not we have to do, be, or have something in order to be valuable. Do we need to succeed to be of value? Do we need to own something to be valuable? Do we need to have a particular title such as CEO, doctor, or Mother in order to feel valued? One of the biggest challenges we may have is seeing our personal self-value as inherent and unconditional.

When we get caught up on the conditional side of the continuum, we fall into a trap or cycle that we constantly have to do something in order to feel valuable, whether that be a getting a university degree, performing in a sport, or having a partner. These can often give us hidden motivations behind why we may be with someone whom we really don't want to be with, but without them we would not feel valuable. In short, conditional esteem is a lie we tell ourselves, which we picked up in the early years of life. We may have been celebrated and given attention when we succeeded in school or beat an opposing team. Because of this, we created meaning structures that taught us that when we do those things, we are valuable and without them, we are nothing. Where this becomes an issue with our health is when we constantly have a need to go harder and harder or that if we don't see constant results in our training, then we are inherently broken or faulty. We could also then look for esteem from others and pursue doing what other people may find valuable so that they tell us how good we are doing. This would also become a cluster with external authority as we are still looking for approval from an authority figure to know that we are valuable.

Conclusion: nobody gets to decide your worth but you. Not even me, who just told you to decide to be valuable. Ironic, isn't it? In all seriousness, when we put conditions on our value we not only lie to ourselves and the next generation who are watching us but we also put ourselves in a constant bind to have to do or be something in order to feel valuable. This presupposes we are working from a space of worthlessness. Our worth as a human being is innate; it is our meaning structures and programs that get in the way of it. This is why we don't have to become more, but rather becoming less can often be the solution, to unbecome what we are not, to unbecome the lies we have told ourselves. Some people are concerned that if they don't have to do something to feel valuable, then they will end up lazy, unmotivated, and unsuccessful, so they end up keeping to these conditions as they serve them and drive them, even if they feel yucky the whole time. The truth is when we work from a place of being worthy and of value, we are working from a place of abundance. We constantly want to give to others because we don't need to do it for validation or worth anymore; we get to do it because it fuels our purpose, not our ego.

Practice: Most thinking patterns are quite neutral, none better nor worse than others. It is harder to argue that with this one. This is an overarching thinking pattern that can really impact all the other programs. The goal here is to find any conditions that we put on our self-worth and to really test them out, see how true they are. If you feel strongly about having to do a particular thing or achieve a particular thing, then maybe it is pointing to a condition you have on your worth. This can be hard to acknowledge, but doing so can set you free. Once you have acknowledged that it is a condition, it is worth asking yourself questions to test why it is so important to you. Here are some suggestions: If they didn't think of me in a particular way, would that really impact my life long term? If I didn't get this job, am I really not worthy of love? What is another belief I could have that serves me better than the one I am running now?

6. Relationship Pattern
Matching and Mismatching

Often when we talk about relationships it is easy to think of a marital or boyfriend/girlfriend type relationship. "Relationship" simply refers to relating to another and the constant dynamics of that relating. Matching and mismatching can be described as looking for sameness (matching) and looking for difference (mismatching). Once again there are deeper reasons why we may either match or mismatch and of course it is contextual. People who have either one of these as a driver will often be completely unaware that they are either continually disagreeing with people or, on the flipside, continually agreeing with people (even when they don't).

When it comes to following a training program or learning a skill, it pays to be a matcher. What this means is that you will do what you can to make sure you match either the program or the person teaching the skill. I considered writing all these programs and the Enneagrams as if I was talking to the person who really leaned into those traits. Although I decided against doing that, I will do it here: mismatchers will look for ways to prove all the information and insight I am sharing wrong, and all power to them. You were never going to agree with me anyway. As for you matchers, you are just hungry for more and more information. Keep that hunger with you in life; it will pay dividends.

Conclusion: matching and mismatching is one of the easiest programs to spot. Mismatchers are the easiest to spot as well; they are the persons who even when they agree with you, will take a different point of view, say something that you may be missing, and even say no when they want to say yes. There is benefit to both viewpoints. If you need someone do a safety inspection of the house you just built, it will pay to have a mismatcher. They will go over it to find all of things that may be an issue. A matcher, however, may be too interested in matching your energy, your tonality, complimenting you on such a nice house. They would better suit the role of the sales agent. As for health, it pays to mismatch and look for difference. That doesn't mean always err on that side. It means to have a critical eye (and mind) in regard to the information you are reading, even what I have shared. It is when either of these ends of the spectrum becomes a driver that it can start to really impact our life and health. Stepping back and having the flexibility to match or mismatch on demand is true personal power.

Practice: if you continually catch yourself matching other people and being agreeable then it is worth leaning into looking at where they are wrong or missing something. This can help bring a healthy level of cynicism to a conversation and a relationship. People who match too much struggle to make up their own mind and often match the status quo. Mismatchers, however, detest the status quo, and although this is often how all innovation and entrepreneurship arise, it really counts to lean into matching and to learn to hear those around you and what input they have without shutting it down straight away. For our health, this means following a training program, trusting, and seeing a nutrition program through to the end and being patient when learning a new skill that is being taught to you by someone you have given your time and money to.

7. Scenario Pattern
Pessimism or Optimism

This pattern can also be known as worst-case and best-case scenario thinking. People may gravitate toward thinking that pessimism or worst-case scenario thinking is negative and not useful, which, would be a very pessimistic way to view pessimism, don't you think?

Once again, both pessimism and optimism have their uses and can be resourceful depending on the context. Too much worst-case thinking can cause someone to freeze and never take action, to neglect the possibilities of their potential and stay stagnant out of fear of "worst" case possibilities. On the flip side, when best case thinking is a driver, the person can become naive and fall victim to the "everything will be fine" way of thinking and become even less responsible for their actions. They may struggle to look at the whole spectrum of possibilities and jump from one thing to the next because of how good the best-case scenario looks. Both sides of the pattern have their utility. For example, if you are wanting to make a change to your health and fitness, being able to consider the best possibility can help get you motivated to making that change. On the flipside, I know a story where a son was brought to his mother, and the father claimed the boy must be really tired; the mother said he wasn't sleeping and that he was unconscious. The father disagreed. The only reason that kid was able to blow out the candles at his next birthday was mainly due to his mother's worst-case scenario thinking.

Conclusion: as with all the patterns, the way that we use these rather than are used by these matters. If either one is a driver, then we no longer are making decisions or thinking clearly as our thinking is clouded by the filter of either pessimism or optimism. Both are actually judgments and are usually future orientated. What this means is that we can get caught up with future potential issues or possibilities that take away from our ability to react to the now based on a filter we didn't even know we were running. When it comes to health, being optimistic is super helpful. Running a healthy level of pessimism will also allow you to check over things, not rush into things and look for mistakes in systems.

Practice: The first step is to catch yourself leaning into either side of the pattern. When you are able to catch yourself leaning into either the worst-case or the best-case scenario, question what the other side would look like. Often worst-case scenario thinking is called dramatizing. Either way, if you catch yourself running this particular pattern, stop and ask yourself what the other end of the scale would look, sound, and feel like. Opening up our awareness to the other side of the spectrum literally allows us to open up our outlook on life. Once we are able to see the wide variety of possibilities, it is important to remind ourselves that these are all just possibilities and that the chances of either extreme occurring is so small. Knowing that, park it and actually deal with reality rather than thinking about it.

8. Emotional Pattern
Unidirectional or Multidirectional

This thinking pattern speaks very much to how well we are able to control our emotions, not just our responses to things but as to whether we allow emotions to spill over to other situations and/ or people. A perfect example of this is when somebody is on a diet, and they have a lunch that isn't planned and maybe it has an extra wine and some chips, and so they have "fallen off the bandwagon." How does this person handle this situation? Is it a one off and will they just go back to the plan or will it fuck up the whole day or maybe even week? Someone who is unidirectional will simply move on. Let it be what it was. Someone who runs more of a multidirectional pattern is likely to let it ruin the day and possible even their diet.

A good indication of this is also whether we allow our emotional response that we have to not being able to do an exercise impact the rest of the session. What about outside of the gym? What about in our relationships? Do we let the fact that we were cut off in traffic impact the way we deal with the barista once we get to work? Do we let this impact how we deal with our work at work? Does that then impact the time we leave and whether or not it becomes "one of those days?"

Unidirectional means that we keep our emotional response to something to just that one thing. We don't drag it across to other parts of our life. Being multidirectional means that our emotional response becomes a state that permeates other areas of our lives.

Conclusion: when we bring awareness to our emotional response and how we are reacting or choosing to respond to a particular situation, we have a choice on whether or not that is going to impact the way we deal with other things. If we truly want to lean into our potential, then learning to leave our issues and emotional responses where they are is one of the most powerful things we can do. This means that we can truly respond to each moment fresh without the baggage of the past, even if it was only a few short minutes ago. It sounds like allowing emotional responses to carry over to other areas of your life may be a negative trait. What if that emotion was happiness? Would that be so bad? Smiling from ear to ear? What if you smiled from ear to ear at a funeral? Maybe that isn't such a bad thing. It is all contextual. The real power here is leaving the so-called negative shit where it belongs: in the past.

Practice: This one can be a tough one. It takes a lot of conscious practice to truly master the ability to learn to let things go in the moment. To learn how to control our emotional response to not poison our mood is really challenging. It takes patience and time and conscious awareness. The key here is learning to detach yourself from what is upsetting you. To look at it from all angles and to ask, is it serving me in this moment? If it isn't, then give yourself 10 seconds or a minute (or really as much time as you need) to breathe deep into your stomach and bring yourself back to the present moment. It takes practice and lots of patience.

9. Timeline Pattern
Static or Process

One of the best ways to look at this type of pattern is to consider whether we see failure as something that is permanent or something that is just part of a process. Do we think that when we get somewhere, that will make us a success or do we see that place as being just a stage in our life as we move through our lives with purpose.

The real importance of this pattern when it comes to our health is whether we are able to see that health is a forever-changing process or it is simply something that we have or do not have. For example,

"All my family is overweight; it is hereditary."
"I wasn't born a runner."
"I am uncoordinated."

This static identity is extremely different to the process mind-set of

"I want to break the cycle so that my kids don't have weight problems."
"I don't find running easy yet, but I am willing to learn."
"Coordination hasn't been my best skill in the past, but I am keen to improve it."

Conclusion: The ability to see things as a process allows us to take a step back and realize that not everything bad that happens is bad and not everything good that happens ends up good. Because nothing ends. When we can understand this, we cease to be frustrated by things that we just don't have control over. Failure is part of the process. Success is a part of the process. Pain is part of the process. Pleasure is part of the process. It is all a process.

Practice: one of the most important practices with this one is to really catch any thoughts or beliefs that you have that are static and potentially stagnant. One of the biggest changes anyone can make to change a static belief into a process statement is to add the word "yet" to the end. That turns "I can't do this" into "I can't do this yet." And that makes all the difference.

10. Motivation Pattern
Motivation Toward or Motivation Away

I remember that when I was about 18, I heard Tony Robbins talk about motivation toward pleasure or motivation away from pain. He went on to say that most of us are motivated to avoid pain rather than to gain pleasure. Although there is a relatively large majority of us who may be motivated by pleasure and what we will gain, for a lot of people things have to get worse before they can make them better. Well, so we think.

The reality is that when we can define a meaningful goal and then not only build pain to not achieving it but also increase the pleasure we would get from achieving it, then the likelihood of achieving that goal increases significantly. It is the integration of both pain and pleasure that gives us meaning to move toward something and meaning to move away from where we are. When we prescribe to just one school of thought, we dramatically cut down our chances of getting clear on why we want to achieve what we want to achieve.

For example:

The goal is to lose 20 kg and regain my body confidence. Fair goal on face value.

What will I gain from it? The extra fitness will allow me to play with my children and participate in their social sports programs, build more confidence in what my body is capable of, and last longer in the bedroom (or at least go for round two)!

What happens if I don't achieve it? I will stay in the same spiral I am now that keeps me from really fully showing up in the world and participating in life fully. I fear that this will become the example I set for my children and that they too will have to take medication that a healthy lifestyle could prevent.

Conclusion: Developing both sides of this pattern can be one of the biggest differences to achieving what we want to achieve. Some struggle with getting clear on what they want and more importantly why it is important to them while others are so far that way inclined that there never is enough pain for them to get going. Those types are dreamers and there is nothing wrong with dreamers, but when dreamers only dream, they stay asleep.

Practice: Start by asking yourself the two questions in the description. See which response lacks emotional pull or push and work on digging deeper there. All the offers I have for you in this book bring their own challenges and remember that what appears hardest for us is often what we need to develop the most.

11. Operational Pattern
Procedures or Options

I have an old business partner, and we used to train together. She would follow her program to a T. I, however, would start my program, swap a couple of exercises to other similar ones I felt like doing, and then often just do a few other extra exercises at the end.

She loved procedures. She was great at following procedures. It is a strength of hers. It wasn't a strength of mine. I liked options. I liked the ability to make a decision in the moment. Some people can eat the same thing day after day and call everyone else lazy or noncommitted. Truth is, they probably just like to have options. This doesn't mean they wouldn't benefit from following procedures; chances are they would. It also doesn't mean that those that follow procedures wouldn't benefit from leaning into options. I have had countless conversations with fully grown adults who are well formally educated and successful in their careers and who tell me how they feel they have wasted their lives because they were too straighty 180. My point here is that once again, developing both sides of this pattern is beneficial.

Options are great when starting an entrepreneurial venture and that program can be the same reason for its downfall. If the entrepreneur isn't able to follow procedures of the systems that run a business, then they will struggle to keep their amazing idea running. But that's okay, they will have plenty more ideas. Of course they will, they love options.

Conclusion: When it comes to health the ability to lean into both sides can be beneficial. It allows us to be disciplined and follow a plan and find opportunities to lean into new experiences that life throws our way, whether that be in the gym for a new class, sticking to a program or nutrition plan, or being part of a multisport social team.

Practice: As a recovering options junkie, I have found that being patient with myself and trusting the process (or procedure) and catching myself wanting to change things and leaning into the opposite of my habitual response powerful. The opposite is much the same. If you find that you are a creature of habit and order the same thing from the menu, take the same hike or the same walk then is then how do you know you wouldn't enjoy a different meal or hike any better unless you try?

12. Self-Confidence Pattern
Low or High

The beauty and tragedy of all these patterns is that they are contextual. Not all of them are drivers. What this means here is that someone may consider themselves to have overall low self-confidence. An absolute large majority of those people will have a skill or a trait that they have high confidence in. What this shows is that they are able to have high confidence; they just have to be confident in their ability to execute that skill. For example, someone may have low confidence in the gym but high confidence when it comes to playing an instrument. What was the skill set and the process for them to build that confidence? Were they patient with themselves? Where they confident when the first started? At one point did they become confident? Did it happen overnight? If not, when?

All these questions are pointing to the fact that we have the ability to become confident of ourselves in any area of our lives. This level of confidence is not to be mistaken by false bravado or an inflated ego. Confidence literally stems from the word *confidere*, which means to have full trust. So to have self-confidence is to have full trust in ourselves.

We may have low confidence in our ability or a skill but high confidence in our ability to learn it. That's the difference. If we bring high confidence to a skill that we have low ability in, this is bravado. If we bring high confidence in ourselves to the learning of the skill, this is the game changer.

Conclusion: Low confidence in ability is fine; remember it is all a process. Bringing high confidence to the skill of learning and to your self is one of the most powerful and transformational things you can do for you and your life.

Practice: To practice self-confidence we have to practice self-trust. We have to trust that we are okay, inherently valuable, and have the will to learn anything. Like all patterns, this can take time. But somewhere along that journey something changes; you may notice it or you may not. You may wake up different one day or you may be completely unaware of when things changed. The key here is to take one step at a time. Pick something you want to develop, be it a skill, a language, talking to the opposite sex, saying sorry, downhill mountain biking, whatever it is, and bring a high level of trust and a high level of confidence in your ability to learn the said skill. Everyone is a beginner at some point.

13. Responsibility Pattern
Less, Too Much, or Healthy Responsibility

One of the major issues that the industry feeds and one that I highlighted earlier in this book is the lack of responsibility on the part of a lot of clients and the overwhelming amount of responsibility on the part of a lot of self-proclaimed coaches. Responsibility refers to our ability to respond. When we are overly responsible for someone else, we take away some of their personal power and ability to respond. We call this helping, and it may yield a short-term result. Long term, it feeds the issue they tried to address in the first place.

It is not possible to be overly responsible somewhere without being under responsible somewhere else. The easiest example of this is when we try and fix other people's problems. Often it is easier to fix their problems than it is to deal with us. That is, in the short term, it is easier to be response able for their issues while we ignore ours.

Healthy responsibility is when we look at each situation and take personal responsibility for what is within our power and allow other people to step up and do the same. This can be some of the most frustrating moments in our lives but can help people who are closest to us the most. Maybe you lean into less responsibility, maybe you lean into more responsibility. Maybe it is a driver for you, maybe it is contextual. Either way, opening our eyes up to this pattern can be one of the most fundamental growth spurts of our life or someone else's.

Conclusion: developing a healthy level of responsibility in your life can free you from carrying everyone else's problems and simultaneously propel you into dealing with yours. Maybe one of yours that you have been less responsible with is how much of other people's problems you have been taking on. Maybe you have been avoiding responding to something that impacts your energy while simultaneously being overly responsible for their issues. Either way finding balance in this pattern is powerful and life changing. Not everyone around you may like it, but that isn't your responsibility either.

Practice: The practice for this one can be tough. One of the key things is to really notice when you are not taking responsibility for areas of your health and your happiness and you are handing that over to someone or something else to take care of. This could come down to conditions we put on our happiness such as waiting for a text message from some in the morning to doing everything for your clients in the gym and calling it service. You aren't servicing them, you're making them codependent on you, and in the long run, that doesn't serve anyone.

14. Persistence Pattern
Patient or Impatient

Initially, this pattern could be perceived to be pretty one sided. Dealing with impatient people may be up there with one of the most frustrating experiences we could go through. Besides, patience is a virtue, right?

Not all the time.

Go back to our example earlier about the mother and her son who was limp. It would be fair to argue that a decent level of impatience would be beneficial in getting him to the hospital in time to save his life. Once again, patience and impatience is contextual. Impatience allows us to keep moving forward and pursue our goals. Patience allows us to be kind to ourselves throughout the process and, consequently, when we are patient with people on their journey, we can help teach them to be patient and love themselves through their own frustrating fallibility.

Conclusion: When we bring patience to ourselves, we have the power to slow down time. We can truly start to take a bit of pressure off ourselves in order to master the task at hand. By contrast, having deadlines and leaning into a little bit of impatience can be so valuable to reaching a result. There are some things we just can't rush, and, often, by trying to rush them, we only rush our frustration to the surface.

Practice: The key offer here is to recognize when we start to put a lot of pressure on ourselves to have things done by a particular time or make comments to ourselves such as "I should know this by now." This type of thinking was learned and most likely served us at some point in our lives; sometimes it served us very well. We have to ask ourselves, is it still serving us today? Or is it slowly eroding away at our soul? Patience is the only antidote. On the flipside, if you are someone who is constantly patient with everyone, this might make you seem like the "nice guy/girl" when in reality people may be taking advantage of that and walking all over you. Sometimes knowingly. Either way, a healthy level of impatience can bring balance to your health and your relationships.

15. Scale Pattern
Black and White–Continuum–Multidimensional
The way that we classify information varies massively throughout these three types. Black-and-white thinking will give people the idea that everything is either this or that. Those are the two options. They will struggle to see things in the gray. You're either in or you're out. Although this type of thinking can help us come to a decision, it can also heavily limit us to seeing everything as binary. Overdone, this can promote an all-or-nothing attitude that very often becomes problematic.

Continuum thinking allows us to see the degrees as we start to see the grayness of the black-and-white options. It turns two options into a multitude of possibilities and opens up our experience to life. For example, when it comes to health, we may initially consider that there is only one real way to train to get strong. Over time, we may start to not only respect but also integrate different methodologies into our own training that we maybe once rejected. Therefore, diehard powerlifters may start to integrate other methodologies into their training as they start to broaden their awareness of what strength really means to them.

Multidimensional thinking starts to truly lean into integration of everything. We start to see how when we are healthy in our mental lives, we become healthier in our physical lives and more productive at work. It truly recognizes how everything impacts everything else and sees relationships between things that, on face value, appear to be worlds apart.

Conclusion: When we move into multidimensional thinking, we truly start to integrate black-and-white thinking and continuum thinking across all areas of our life. This means we are able to see the importance of rest and how that plays a role in our relationship. It means we can see all of the possibilities and then cut them down to make the best decision in that moment. It means we can think laterally about how when we take responsibility for our mental and physical health, it does actually impact those around us and the next generation.

Practice: See if you find yourself either becoming dogmatic about the right answer (black and white) or indecisive because you see so many possibilities you definitely couldn't pick the right one. Either extreme is unresourceful. When integrated with a healthy level of multidimensional thinking, we can truly start to see how our behaviors, actions, and personal responsibility make a significantly larger impact than we may have originally thought.

* * *

Too many men try to master the world because it is easier than mastering ourselves. The continual development of our own self-mastery is a noble quest, and I would argue a necessary one. This path can be one of the hardest, but understanding it can make the developments made in the other two areas of health (movement and nutrition) significantly easier.

There is a story about the knights of the round table that Joseph Campbell is famously renowned for sharing with the world. It is an excerpt from a novel written about the Holy Grail by an anonymous 13th-century monk. Joseph believes this best conveys the human experience.

King Arthur and his noble knights are seated at the round table, and the Holy Grail appears before them, covered in a great, radiant cloth. And then all of a sudden, it disappears. Gawain, who is Arthur's nephew, suggests a quest to discover the Holy Grail unveiled.

Now we come to the text that interested me. The text reads, "They thought it would be a disgrace to go forth in a group. Each entered the Forest Adventurous at the point he himself had chosen, where it was darkest and there was no way or path."

You enter the forest at the darkest point, where there is no path. Where there is a way or path, it is someone else's path; each human being is a unique phenomenon.

The idea is to find your own pathway to bliss.

PART II

··

The
BODY

··

Move Your Ass

Let's get something straight first. You don't need a gym membership to have a healthy life. A gym membership doesn't make you a better person, and paying a weekly or monthly fee doesn't automatically make you fitter. This is coming from someone who has worked in gyms since he was 15 and owned his own since he was 22. The most fundamental thing that I want you to take from this chapter is that movement helps you to experience life. Outside of the high-level strength sports world, your training really should help improve your life outside of the gym rather than just chasing numbers in the gym. Higher numbers in strength doesn't directly correlate to being able to do more outside the gym. I am a massive advocate of strength training. There comes a point where diminishing returns do occur though. There comes a point where maybe niggles start to kick in, and you have to make more trade-offs to chase higher numbers in the gym. Maybe it isn't higher numbers on your weights, maybe it is faster numbers on your runs. Either way, you have to make a decision as to what you are willing to trade. Is it time away from your family? Are you avoiding something? Do you think the next PR is going to bring you happiness that will last forever? Just like your last PR?

The most important thing is that you move. If your one hour in the gym doesn't positively impact your 23 hours outside of it, then it no longer is an investment; it is a cost.

If you never go to the gym but you go for walks with your spouse and play social tennis, then this can be significantly healthier than people who go to the gym seven days a week. I have already mentioned that some people who exercise that much have a high risk of training for the sake of training away their anxiety.

Add that to a physically tight body from imbalanced training and avoiding addressing other difficulties in our lives such as relationships, and someone who looks healthy on Instagram selling diet programs isn't so healthy after all.

So in short gyms can be an amazing place where people can transform their lives. They become more than just a gym. They become a second home, a second family, a spiritual experience. When done well, a gym can be an integral part of personal development, mind, body, and heart.

Over the coming chapter, I will be offering plenty of ideas for different training options. Although most of my experience is in training, I have reached a part in my career where after training literally thousands of people I have come to the realization that what's most important is that you are having fun and challenging yourself around a group of people who are doing the exact same thing. There is no type of training that is better than the rest. There are too many factors. Of course powerlifting is better for overall strength than marathon running. But outside of those obvious options, it comes down to what you enjoy and what you want to work toward.

If I was to cover the three most important factors to training to simplify it, they would be the following:

1. Choose something aligned with your goals

This may sound obvious, but it really is rule number one. The problem for most people is that they aren't clear on their goals. They stick with just weight loss or tone up. They lack the other important goals of being mentally stimulated, challenged, being around a group of people going in the same direction, being a part of something bigger than themselves, having fun. Get real and get deep with your goals and think about what you really want out of your training. Physical results, social dynamics, life PRs, all of it. When you can get clear on this you can get clear on what is important to you when considering a training program. Fuzzy goals yield fuzzy results so don't just leave it at weight loss, you can lose weight at a hospital.

2. Something you can do long term

One of the biggest factors that I have seen stop people from achieving long-term results is that they go into their training as if it were a 12-week challenge where they restrict themselves unrealistically while hating themselves and secretly telling themselves that the physical results and emotional response from seeing a number on the scales will be worth it. Then when they get there, they will just maintain it. which often means to go back to an old lifestyle. Imagine doing this with any other part of your life such as work. I am going to work my ass off for 12 weeks and then just work to maintain after that. It sounds ridiculous, because it is. If you want long-term change, change long term. In most cases, the training has to be sustainable on the body; you have to enjoy the training as well. Enjoying the training doesn't necessarily mean you have to be excited to do burpees; it may mean you enjoy the challenge of the workout, maybe it means you enjoy the people and working together. Either way, if you don't enjoy it, it won't last.

3. Actively learn along the way

For real long-term sustainable change we must learn along the way. This is the whole point of the book, continual education to help improve our HIQ so that we can keep the results we gain. If we have short-term physical improvements but without long-term mental improvements, then at some point, we will balance out and return to our default HIQ. Find a trainer, YouTube channel, gym, or coach who will help educate you along the journey. Ask as many questions as you can. Take full responsibility for your health and your learning. That is how you turn any money you spend on your health into a true investment. This will help you change your life, inspire the people around you, and lead the next generation. Actively learn along the way.

The HIQ Move Map

The movement map was the first component of the HIQ Map to be established. I used this in my gyms to help coach coaches to coach movement. It is the same framework we use for programming, exercise selection, and even building a community.

The three levels of the Move Map are

- Safe
- Strong
- Sexy

The reason why I went with move rather than exercise is because exercise is a compartment of movement rather than the other way around. Some people never need to set foot in a gym or have an "exercise" routine, and they are happy just as they are. Why should I suggest any changes? If they don't have a problem or desire anything different then nothing needs to change. At least not in their world.

Although I am an advocate for a healthy level of gym training, I hope I have driven home the point here that the gym isn't the solution for everyone. It can be part of the solution for some but for some people, buying a puppy and taking it on daily walks yields the happiness and level of exercise that they are seeking. It all comes down to our true goals.

This also feeds into the start of the HIQ Move Map that begins by looking at the safe stage. So before discussing training options and offers, let's take a look at each stage and what they represent.

Safe

Some trends in the fitness industry are unconsciously encouraging short-term amateur athletes, and in doing so they are consequently sacrificing long-term freedom of movement. One of the key elements of any fitness program or sport for that matter is moving safely. This stage is about building spatial awareness and body intelligence. For a lot of us, we have to really learn where we are in space in order to be able to instruct this meat skeleton to do what we want it to do. When exercising it is common to fall into the trap of focusing on the objective goal. That is, move this bar from point A to point B as many times as you can. This then brings out the technique of the Nazis. I have one problem with the technique though; it is incomplete. People have different body shapes and lever lengths. They have different training ages, different jobs, and different training and movement history, not to mention different learning preferences, different personality traits, and different personal challenges. So technique is not a bad concept for guidelines, but as both coaches/trainers and athletes/ clients, we must see technique as an individual variation and process of those guidelines.

The majority of us aren't getting paid to exercise; we don't because it enhances our life. So be careful sacrificing that enhancement long term to chase short-term satisfaction. Play the long game; you have your body and your whole life (hopefully). Take the time to learn and develop movement. At my gym Functional Fitness Australia, we don't teach technique, we help develop movement. That is my offer for you.

What does it mean to move safely with body intelligence? When coaching coaches I ask them a few questions;

1. Are they able to move with stability?
2. Do they have a healthy range of motion while they maintain stability?
3. Can they repeat that range of motion with that stability and under fatigue?

These questions, although they are more like standards of movement, can be applied to all the different types of sports and fitness endeavors. From tennis, to weightlifting to gymnastics to rock climbing.

When looking at exercise selection for gym training, we want to be able to ask similar questions that relate to the individual. What this means is simple and basic work. It can keep programs safe and effective. The majority of people who want to be able to go on hikes, play social sport, play with their kids, be pain free, and feel confident in their bodies just don't need to snatch barbells and do handstands and run super-long distances. This doesn't mean I am against any of these movements or options in particular; this is simply looking at the safe parameters for people who are wanting to maximize the most in life and minimize potential risks in the gym. Twenty percent of the exercises will yield 80 percent of the results people need. The problem can come when the other 80 percent of exercises are thrown in and the base 20 percent is ignored. Get the fundamentals drilled in for years. Don't practice something until you get it right; practice until you can't get it wrong.

Like all levels of the HIQ Map, when progressing from here to strong we want to transcend and include these principles. When moving to higher levels in the Move Map we don't want to neglect the safety precautions. When we learn new skills and more complex expertise, we want to be able to go back and treat these skills with the same eye for detail as we did the fundamental skills. When we level up, we don't lose the basics; we continue to develop them.

Benchmarks for the Safe Stage

The safe stage is for anyone starting out in a particular area. One of the ways to consider where we are in the Move Map is to think of it in terms of our training age. Our training age is an amalgamation of your training history or experience and your detail to that training. For example, 15 years of ineffective training would likely yield a younger training age than someone who has been training for 5 years under highly qualified supervision. The former is more likely to be 1 year of experience done 15 times. It is important to know that it doesn't matter what industry you are in, that is not 15 years' experience. It is one.

The interesting thing when it comes to training is that we could potentially be at a training age of say 10 years as a high-level competitive cyclist and therefore have climbed to a mastery level in movement. However, when we switch codes to powerlifting we start out at a safe level again. One way to think about this is to consider that this person's training has helped develop so many critical skills and body intelligence; however, at no point does this person put a weighted barbell on their back and squat to find their one repetition max. Cyclists are concentric athletes and are constantly reinforcing a flexed spine in an approximately 45-degree hip-hinged position. What this means is that they are always pushing with their legs and never load their legs and spine to move through a bilateral (two feet at once) eccentric (contacting but lowering) movement like a squat. Their body simply is not yet ready to go where the mind has gone for the past 10 years.

They have to go through all the standards of safe to be able to develop the movement patterns, build sensory awareness through range, and bring stability to that range. If they don't do this, it will almost certainly cause some issues down the track.

Questions that go into considering our training age:

- How long have you been training in a specific style?
- Do you have experience in other training that carries over?
- What is your attention to detail out of 10 when you train? (0 being a low level and 10 being high level)

These three questions can allow us to gauge where we are at with our level on the Move Map. The standards of each stage actually vary depending on what you want to get out of it. For safe, it is really about building a connection to the physical body and knowing where our body is in space. The fundamentals for powerlifting, gymnastics, or being a triathlete vary from discipline to discipline. However moving safely and building your training age is crucial no matter what the discipline.

A training age under 400 hours in any particular discipline would be generally considered safe. This would take approximately two years of deliberate practice at just under four hours a week. Brainless exercising does not count; it is conscious practice of the actual skills and required detail. For some people, it may be 12 to 18 months. For others it could be three to four years.

Benchmarks:

- **Eager and keen to learn and go all in.**
- **Gets "newbie" gains, which is often just neural adaptations. This means they learn how to do things easier.**
- **Less than 400 hours of deliberate practice.**
- **Focus mainly on performance and not the integrated and holistic approach for their whole life.**

Strong

The strong stage transcends just understanding the physical components of movement and body intelligence. It takes all the safe standards into account and adds another dynamic. In this stage, people really start to develop a deeper connection with their bodies and start to see how different areas of their life affect their performance. Although strong can be a reference to building strength, what it really refers to is having a strong bond or relationship with our bodies. At this level we truly start to understand that everything is connected. You start to see how a strong mind-set won't get you through weeks of bad sleep and training your ass off. That strong mind-set becomes a weakness as the body doesn't recover well enough to be able to perform again. Although that strong mind-set may have served you in other areas of your life, our strengths at extremes can also become a weakness.

At this stage we start to understand that training isn't always exercise. We start to taper our training throughout the week and over the year to make sure that our body gets adequate recovery for it to perform. This stage is where we start to truly understand the relationship the body has with all the areas of our lives. Signs of earlier stages are when people get frustrated with not lifting the same amount of weight as they did the week before without realizing they have an assignment due at school; work is stressful, they are experiencing a rough patch with their partner, and are lacking sleep compared to normal. At the strong stage, people start to see all this as one whole rather than separate parts, and they change their training accordingly. They may reduce the intensity or the number of sessions or maybe even take a week off. They see the big picture rather than the need to smash the gym every day and get gains week by week.

No one can do that. Unless you are Ed Coan. (Feel free to google him)

Benchmarks for the Strong Stage

People at this stage appear to take pressure off themselves and relax with their training a little more. To an unaware mind it may look like they are falling off the bandwagon when in reality, they are giving themselves space to see the big picture. In doing so, they actually pull more meaning to their training, and as a result their training will have a deeper why, a more sustainable approach, and yield a long-term progression. In this space the person is more interested in how their training is positively impacting their life rather than just chasing numbers. Surprisingly enough this is often what they need in order for their numbers to increase. Prior to this they may have been overtraining and under-recovering, and therefore simply weren't performing. This type of "burnout" actually encourages them to step back and revaluate why they do it. Like magic, when they take away the frustration and pressure they start to once again get improvements in the gym. This can often remind us not to take it too seriously. People at this stage start to take more personal responsibility for their own education about their bodies and what they need to recover and feel good. Remember this is often after the person has completed about 400 hours of deliberate practice.

This person's training age will often be somewhere between 400 and 10,000 hours of deliberate practice. Although there is a massive gap between 400 and 10,000 hours, the reason is because it takes blood, sweat, and years to develop this stage. A lot of people stay at this stage. They may be here for 20, 30, or even 40 years, and there is nothing wrong with that; it is perfectly fine and absolutely sustainable. One of the key things about mastering anything that we want is that at some point we stop counting the hours. We stop getting caught up in wanting the black belt, and we just start doing the work required. That's when you know someone is deep in their strong stage and are building a deeper purpose to something that becomes more than just a lifelong, sustainable approach to health. This happens at a later stage of strong as they transition into sexy. And as this person transitions from strong into sexy their impact starts to become intergenerational. They start to inspire not just their generation but the generation below them.

Benchmarks:

- **More than 400 hours of deliberate practice but less than 10,000.**
- **Start to look at their training in a more holistic and integrated way.**
- **Their "gains" slow down, but their learning doesn't and in most cases, it increases.**
- **Have a more sustainable approach to their training and health to avoid burnout and preventable injuries.**

Sexy

Sexy is truly movement mastery. This is the black belt of the physical domain. Sometimes literally. The interesting thing about this level is that it is often so niche or in just one domain. Most of the training at a safe level for general life is called general physical preparedness or GPP. At the sexy stage it is movement mastery and often of one specific skill. For example, the skill could be gymnastics, weightlifting, golf, or even Brazilian jiujitsu. They may have a broad base across other sports or have skills that could carry across other domains; however, this is the particular domain in which they have approached movement mastery.

At this stage people start to have their type of movement integrated into their daily lifestyle and often spend their time developing, thinking, and practicing these skills every day in some form or another for years. If they aren't physically practicing they are reading about it; if they aren't reading about it, they are teaching it, if they aren't teaching it, they are watching videos on it; if they aren't watching videos on it, they are dreaming about it.

For people at this stage, discipline is just a way of life. So much so that sometimes you may not even know that they are so competent at it. Often it is other people who will tell you about their achievements or skills. Make no mistake; it takes years and more often than not decades to get to this stage. You cannot rush this stage; you cannot buy your way to this stage. This is a lifelong process of learning how to get in flow, being present, and being connected in body, mind, and soul.

The reason why this is called sexy is because how effortless these people make their chosen skill set look. They often make it look so incredibly easy and smooth when in reality they are constantly moments away from disaster. That's what makes it so heroic. It is these people who push the human limits, who show us what is truly possible. That's why we stand in awe of them; that's why we clap and pay money to watch them. They are showing us glimpses of the human potential we all harness. And even though it looks effortless, deep down we all know that an immeasurable amount of work went into that moment, that skill set, with hundreds, if not thousands of stumbles along the way. But the majority of us sit back and admire the tenacity, the lunacy, to go after the impossible. That's why it is called sexy.

Benchmarks for the Sexy Stage
People at this stage are usually in the "black belt" category of their chosen field. More often than not they are also teachers. The people at the higher stages of sexy are masters and teachers and have also developed leadership skills that make their mark intergenerational rather than simply a good exercise program. People at the highest levels talk about how when they are in flow, it is the most spiritual experience they have experienced. What they are pointing to is the times in their life everything slowed down and they were fully present to the moment, what was required of that moment, and their ability to perform in that moment.

One of the biggest differences for people here is their desire to give back to the discipline that gave them so much. They become an inspiration for people around them and are more often than not extremely humble. They see their work as a form of art expressed physically, and their passion becomes infectious to those who spend time with them. The majority of the population may never get here in a physical domain. We may reach this in a parental domain, maybe in our career. Either way, not everyone needs to be here. The point of having the sexy stage is not so that everyone transcends to such a high level metaphysically but rather we operate our training and integrate our mind and soul into everything we do so that we can live the life we want and offer the next generation the exact same thing. Sexy isn't for everyone, but in a way it is. When someone is in this space and they're in their element, we can't help but watch in awe.

The sexy benchmarks can almost appear like they are too hazy or vague, but those that are there completely understand.

Benchmarks:

- **They stopped counting hours but somewhere over the 10,000 mark.**
- **They don't train, they study art physically, mentally and spiritually.**
- **They measure their improvements by the amount of lives they impact.**
- **Their discipline is an expression of them and vice versa.**

Training Styles

I don't have the perfect training plan for everyone. Like I mentioned earlier, people need to have their own personal variation if they really want to further develop both their physical body and their HIQ.

That being said, I decided to focus on three types of strength and fitness training: strength training, functional fitness and aerobic training. Under each type I have attempted to break down the pros and cons that each style offers.

My offer for you is to find something that interests you that you may want to pursue further. You can find further training programs at www.bossfit.online.

Please also note that these training styles aren't taking into account activities like social sport, running clubs, and surfing among many, many others. These are simply offers for some different styles that may help you move closer toward your goals outlined earlier in the book.

The training styles are broken down into three categories: strength, functional fitness, and cardiovascular. I have chosen 10 options and offered pros and cons for each style. And just in case you missed it the first time, I haven't covered every single training style in this book. I have narrowed it down to approximately 12 for the sake of keeping it short, yet offering options, and to clarify, the training options are in no particular order either.

Enjoy.

Strength Training

Strength can be a hot topic when it comes to what it actually means. To some people it may mean flexibility or the benefits one gains from yoga. To others it could mean the ability to run a full game of football. What I am referring to here is resistance training with the goal of improving the body's physical strength.

Powerlifting

Powerlifting is a sport that consists of three lifts: the bench press, the back squat, and the dead lift. All these movements are completed with a barbell, and in competition there are three attempts at each lift allowed to score a one repetition max in each lift.

Recently, this sport has had a surge thanks to the garage gym movement and fitness companies like CrossFit. For a long time this sport was kind of seen as underground and was only reserved for big guys with big guts who grunted a lot. This stereotype has since been smashed where literally as of the day of this writing there are 55 kg females squatting 260 kg. This is absolutely next level strong. No beards, no fat guts. Just strong, strong people.

There are plenty of local powerlifting clubs around, and although they often have large bearded men there, I have always found them to have a welcoming and a positive environment to be around, the gyms and the bearded men that is. The other thing is that you do not have to compete to train in this discipline. In fact, I would suggest most people who train this way never compete; they just love the benefits from this style of training.

Pros: Build strength, gyms are often communities and supportive, get strong glutes (booty).

Cons: Can be repetitive, don't promote fitness-type exercise, will often get tight, and may restrict joint mobility.

Where: Most places will have local gyms in your neighborhood or nearby. I suggest googling and checking them out. The best

I have come across online is Juggernaut Training Systems (JTS). Find out more at www.jtsstrength.com.

Olympic Lifting

Talk about rising from the ashes. In recent years, much like powerlifting, Olympic lifting has had a resurgence for pretty much the same reasons. Olympic lifting is the lifting you see at the Olympics (thanks Captain Obvious), where competitors complete two lifts the snatch and the clean and jerk.

Learning Olympic lifting has more similarities to learning Brazilian jiujitsu than it does to powerlifting. It is a more dynamic and more demanding on the mobility and flexibility of joints. Lifts are not usually as high however you almost can't compare the two types of lifting.

If you have the patience and desire, then learning Olympic lifting is both an amazing strength training tool and access to a fantastic global community. I have been fortunate enough to train with international level lifters at gyms in different countries, and each time they have been extremely welcoming and a pleasure to train with.

Pros: Building power, increasing mobility of joints, building strength.

Cons: Learning the skill can be extremely frustrating, can become tedious, and it doesn't encourage cross platform training.

Where: Like powerlifting, there can be some great local clubs with tremendous coaches who dedicate their life to lifting and teaching. Failing that, there are some great websites and coaches online to learn from. Once again, I would recommend JTS. They also have cool shirts.

Strongman

Out of all the strength sports, I would argue that strongman/ woman is the most functional. From carrying objects to throwing things and picking up heavy stuff for reps it can be quite the spectacle. The competitions are forever changing, and if you have a strongman/woman coach then your training is likely to vary more than the other two strength sports.

Using equipment such as heavy ass stones, yokes, farmer handles, barbells, and many other outlandish strength tests, they really do test who is the strongest across domains. I personally don't have a lot of experience in strongman competitions although I regard them highly for their feats of strength.

Pros: You get strong, you get really strong, and you eat a lot of burgers.

Cons: You may run out of breath walking up two flights of stairs, you have to buy new pants, and you eat a lot of burgers.

Where: Much the same as above all though due to the fact that there is much more equipment needed the clubs and coaches can be harder to find. Searching online for strongman clubs/gyms in your area is the best bet.

Bodybuilding

You didn't think I was going to leave Arnie out did you? Although I never ventured down the bodybuilding route, and I have my gripe with it for a lot of reasons there are some amazing and inspiring people who live and breathe bodybuilding. Bodybuilding can be your main form of strength training, and failing that, it is a great form of accessory work to supplement your strength training. It is important to note that not everyone that body builds is a bodybuilder.

Bodybuilding can be a safe approach to strength training due to the slow nature of the lifting. This doesn't mean that the others aren't safe, and it can even be argued that slow strength training is less applicable in real life than the other three types of strength training. All that aside, bodybuilding is a fantastic way to either train or supplement your training. It can be great for strengthening tendons and joints with slower, higher rep resistance training than long-term heavy lifting. Most bodybuilding can be done in just about any commercial gym, and I highly recommend you do your due diligence and homework on your coach. Find someone who has extensive knowledge, expertise, and passion.

Pros: Available almost anywhere, simple and easy to get started, can be a mixture of strength training and cardio.

Cons: Can become very self-obsessed on image, can become tedious, with a lot of mixed information on the Internet and in the gym.

Where: Literally almost every single commercial facility. Always do your homework when finding out who to follow

and where to obtain your program. The best bodies on Instagram aren't always the best educators and coaches.

Functional Fitness

Functional fitness has been at the forefront of the recent surge in fitness trends and for good reason too. But, with everything good comes the rest. It is important to make the distinction between functional fitness and functional movement. People can be doing so-called functional fitness exercises in a dysfunctional fashion with no improvement. So can this really be called "functional" fitness? Either way most forms of functional fitness training styles include a strength component and a conditioning or fitness component. It is literally the best of both worlds. Most of these training programs fall under the category mentioned earlier called GPP. For most people wanting to get the most out of their life outside of the gym this would be my general recommendation. My last words on this is that I highly recommend you find a facility or coach that positions themselves as an educator/education facility and not just an exerciser or exercise facility.

GPP Program

My first introduction to this style of training was the Gym Jones. I watched their video on YouTube training the actors of the *300* movie and just wanted to learn about the training style. Most "functional" style gyms will offer their variation of GPP. The most famous example of GPP is CrossFit. Many people were introduced to the garage-gym-type training through CrossFit, and the name owned the space for a very long time. Although it comes with its critics, there are plenty of fantastic coaches in the CrossFit world who can help people reach their potential. The interesting thing about these types of gyms is making sure that you do your homework again. There can be some massive differences between these styles of gyms, and even if they have the same names or similar names, more often than not, the bigger the classes, the less attention to detail you receive. Although a good coach with more clients is often a better coaching experience than a poor coach with less.

I am a big advocate for this style of training; my business is even called Functional Fitness Australia. Like all the others, just do your homework and find a place that suits you. They usually offer free or cheap trials, put their programing online for free, and are more often than not family run.

Pros: Can get you fit, lean, and strong, be a part of a community, to learn about your body and how to take care of it.

Cons: Can become super competitive; classes can sometimes be quite large, with higher price point than a commercial facility.

Where: Functional training is available almost anywhere at the moment. Even the big box gyms have got on board and cleared an area in their gyms for functional training. Once again a web search of your local area will do the trick. Failing that, we have online programming for free at www. funcfitness.com.au that you can follow.

Bodyweight Specialists

There are a number of different options when it comes to bodyweight training. There is everything from strictly gymnastic type training through to parkour. Some people prefer to go for this style of training due to the fact that you don't need any weights and little equipment.

Gymnastic-style training can help get people strong, lean, and more often than not super flexible. It can be great for training around lower-back injuries and other injuries, depending on what they are of course. It is also never too late to start this style of training, and there are so many different ways to scale the movements. You don't need to be able to do a handstand or a pull up to get started.

Pros: Little equipment, can keep people lean and light, can start at any level.

Cons: Can become repetitive; a lot of movements can require a great deal of skill and patience; doesn't have a great deal of carry over to strength sports or fitness.

Where: You can try a local gymnastic club or something similar; otherwise, there are a lot of different coaches online who offer online programming and educational programs. One of the best is gymnastic bodies.

Aerobic

Triathlon/ironman/marathon training

One of the most challenging and cross-aerobic conditioning types of training is the triathlon or ironman-style training. These disciplines can often bring a variety of different challenges and terrains to a type of fitness training where you are constantly pushing yourself. Most triathlon, marathon, and ironman clubs have beginner programs that allow you to get started wherever you are and start out with free programs, running groups, and shorter beginner events.

Although this has never personally been my thing, I have had countless friends and clients go down this path and absolutely love this style of training due to its outdoors nature and that you are able to compete against yourself and your numbers.

Pros: Your fitness level will dramatically increase; you have access to a new community with new events outdoors.

Cons: You may be prone to new injuries if not conditioned, can be weather dependent, and not conducive to building muscle.

Where: Most cities and towns will have running groups and competitions; the best thing again would be to jump on and web search clubs in your local area. Failing that, there is a couch to 5K running program at www.c25k.com that can help get you started.

Obstacle Course Race

Something that has gained massive popularity in recent years has been the obstacle course race (OCR) scene. Nowadays, there are an abundance of options when it comes to OCRs, and these can either be a great event to train up for or something fun to jump into on the weekend.

It is a little bit hard to train specifically for these events as sometimes you won't know what will be on the course until you get there. That and the fact that they can have over 20 obstacles and can be as long as a half marathon. Some world events even go for 24 hours. As extreme as these can get, there are ample opportunities to jump in at a beginner level at just about every event. These events can be as fun or as serious as you want to make them. Put your physical capabilities to the test or grab a friend and pay to run and get muddy.

Pros: Can really test your limits, can be a great event to train for, outdoors and lots of fun.

Cons: Due to the terrain, injuries can be an issue; you will have mud in places you wouldn't believe, weather dependent.

Where: These events happen all year round. Check out Spartan Race, Tough Mudder, and Warrior dash just to name a few. There are heaps!

Boxing and Martial Arts

Without a doubt one of the best types of conditioning is almost any form of combat sport. Now although there is a difference between the boxfit style training and actual boxing training, either way it is a great workout. If you don't like learning how to punch or learning how to defend a punch, then stick to the boxfit stuff. Outside of that I think the whole world could benefit greatly from learning a martial art or to box correctly. Boxing is a different beast to martial arts; however, it heavily depends on the values and quality of the coach.

Learning a combat sport is twofold as it can be an amazing workout but you also learn life skills. I personally have seen these skills help people mature into fine adults and face their fears in the right environment. These skills can also help teach you self-defense skills and build amazing body awareness. Some of my favorite martial arts are Thai kickboxing and Brazilian jiujitsu due to their history, discipline, and effectiveness.

Pros: Build self-confidence and body confidence, learn self-defense, a great workout.

Cons: Probably will get punched in the face, be prone to niggly injuries; dealing with egos can be challenging.

Where: Once again the best thing here is to do your due diligence and search what is nearby.

Read reviews and be clear about what you want to get out of the training. A lot of facilities are now way less intimidating than even just a decade ago and welcome anyone who is keen to learn.

The Physical Bank Account

Something that I haven't stressed too much yet is the importance of recovery. The physical bank account is a metaphor for how we should address our body. There are things we do that withdraw from our physical bank account, such as exercise, lack of sleep, or eating so-called "junk food." There are also things we do to give back to our body that help it recover, such as sleep, active rest, and following a healthy nutritional eating plan.

Most of us don't overexercise; we underrecover. We don't do all the things we could do to allow us to recover to go again and build on our training stimulus. Often as we start to gain momentum with our training, we start training in the gym more and more. In doing so, we often neglect to recover more even though we are going harder than ever before. Sooner or later this will end up sending you down the path you don't want to go down.

So to avoid overexercising and preventable injuries I offer some ideas for recovery. Over time, it is crucial to learn to listen to your body and find out the best recover practices for you. Although we can sometimes just put all exercise stimuli and recovery practices in the physical or objective area of our lives, the truth is quite often things such as meditation, and even ending dramatic and toxic relationships can pay dividends for your physical bank account.

1. Sleep

Who has time for sleep in today's world, huh? Well, if we don't make time for sleep, chances are we will have to make time for the big sleep (the one you don't wake up from) because lack of sleep is one of the biggest factors contributing to obesity and cardiovascular disease. If we aren't getting an adequate amount of sleep each week, then everything suffers, yep, everything, including sex.

2. Mobility

Spending some time to get flexy and sexy isn't such a bad idea when it comes to recovery. This can be a great way to get in tune with your body and release tight muscles that often pull on joints. It doesn't have to be taken to the extreme where you become so flexible it's scary. It is a great way to make use of your down time when listening to some music or watching some television, or during your quiet time. Increasing mobility of joints allows for safer positions and helps release tension in the muscles and tendons that act on those joints. Overall this is one of the easiest things you can do to help prevent injuries and increase performance. If you want some inspiration, then check out www. romwod.com for more routines and options. ROMWOD is set up as a subscription, so if you are after some free tuff then check out mobilitywod on YouTube for heaps of great content.

3. Active rest

This means rest. But be active. Just not too active. So go for a walk. Or a swim. Maybe a round of golf. But in all seriousness, you don't have to do nothing when you rest. Being active when you rest can give you many benefits such as getting outside, circulating blood back through the muscles to aid recovery from nutrient delivery and overall range of movement. At least one day a week should be devoted to some low-intensity active rest that you enjoy.

4. Nutrition

Please see the next chapters for nutrition information.

5. Meditation

Although this is still something I haven't delved super deep into, meditation (or at least quiet personal time) is one of the most impactful things we can do for our mental health. There are multiple different forms of meditation, and once again it is about finding which style feels right for you. There are usually spiritual teachers or the like who are trained to guide people through the process, but if that is not your thing then there are multiple apps such as Smiling Sind, Headspace, and Calm that allow you to do it in the comfort of your own home, and they also help keep you on track. If you are not at a stage where meditation is your thing yet, then by all means finding five to ten minutes a day to sit and focus on your breath is one of the most powerful things you can do.

If you want to get started, then you can start by taking deep breaths into your stomach through your nose and breathing out through your mouth to a 10-breath count. Focus on just your breath and filling your abdomen with as much air as possible as if it was a balloon. Breathing is one of the most powerful calming tools we have because when we focus on it, it brings us back to the present moment. Our thoughts can be about the future, we can have feelings about the past, but our body is always in present.

6. Massage/manual therapy

Getting manual therapy is another form of recovery that can pay dividends for your body. There are multiple different types of therapies to choose from, such as physiotherapy right through to acupuncture or dry needling. Although I have personal preferences, what works for each person and their personal preference will vary. A good chiropractor will be better than a poor or ignorant physio. A fantastic and caring physio will be better than a poorly trained osteopath, and so on.

An integration of all of these is what is highly recommended. Overall, my main point in this section is look after your body; don't just flog it. Some people service their cars more than they do their bodies. The truth is, the body needs servicing too, in more ways than one.

If you want some more information on recovery, then some of the guys at RP Strength have some great content on this subject. Check it out at www.renaissanceperiodization.com/recovering-from-training

The Coaching Commandments

Over the last 15 years, I have collected a number of principles that have helped me connect better as a coach and helped clients and athletes achieve their goals. I put together 15 principles that I call the coaching commandments; they help encapsulate what I have talked about within this chapter as well as expanding further from both a coach and a client/athlete perspective.

This is written in a way to speak to coaches but the principles are for everyone. This is an taken from my e-book available at www.davenixon.com.au.

1 Movement Over Exercise

This commandment is the first one because it shifts from the idea of cookie-cutter technical points to a more individual focus of movement. With things like different lever lengths, different training ages, different jobs, different sports, different goals, and different restrictions, we need to understand that we need different variations of the same movements. What works for one person is not going to always work for the next.

Strip the body of skin, fat, muscles, and imagine you have X-ray vision. Look at the person's posture and structure like this; add the muscular layer and then prescribe what information will be best for them. Broad technical cues that are given to a mass population is just one of the reasons we are seeing injuries we could be easily avoiding. Really focus on ensuring that each individual has their own understanding of what their movement should be rather than trying to force each individual into some prearranged idea of what "technique" should look like.

If people do not move well then simply putting them through poor motor patterns will lead to pain at some stage. Continue to place emphasis on good motor patterns. People are quick to sacrifice good movement for "strength" or "smashing out a workout" in order to get results. The issue with this is that they often sacrifice long-term progression for a quick before and after selfie for a few likes.

Once again, don't practice something until you get it right; practice until you cannot get it wrong.

2 Safety First

At my gym, Functional Fitness Australia, we use a system we designed called safe, strong, sexy.

This system allows us to teach people to first move safely and then develop necessary strength through a particular movement. It is easy to fall into the trap in the fitness industry that increasing the load we lift means we are getting stronger.

There are a couple of issues with this approach.

1. The initial stages often show more increase in weights and therefore a larger increase in "strength."

This isn't always true. In fact, it is rarely true. These are commonly called "newbie gains," and their real name is "neural adaptations."

You are simply learning how to move the weight easier. Your body is adapting to make it more efficient. Easily put, you are learning how to use the strength you already have. When your strength appears to slow down, this is where the real strength gains occur.

It takes months to get fit, years to get strong, and just a moment to get injured. Kind of . . . Injuries often are built up over time. Creep loading on tendons and joints slowly put the joint into a vulnerable position. Or a muscle is continually being overloaded day by day and then in a moment it breaks or something goes "twang"! We think the injury happened there, but chances are it has been happening for months and it reached breaking point there. Most injuries can be avoided by intelligent coaching and awareness-driven training.

2. It does not mean that you are becoming stronger with what is truly important to you outside of the gym. A common misconception is that we should get stronger. But for what? And how strong do we need to be?

Now let's clarify this right now before I go on; I thoroughly do believe strength is a skill and is also a beneficial skill for every single human being. My point isn't that you shouldn't squat or that you shouldn't dead lift. My point is how much do you need to fuel your life outside of the gym?

How many clients do you think are executing their coaches'/trainers' goals and not actually their goals? That's why I ask, how strong is strong enough? Right now in the industry we are seeing A LOT of people sacrificing long-term movement for short-term strength.

For what?

I have some friends who lift some serious loads of weight. They dead lift and squat in excess of 300 kg and they love it. I am not talking about these people. I am talking about Gerry the accountant, who has to go back to work and sit down for nine hours, garden for four hours on Sunday, and genuinely wants to kick the soccer ball with his kids. What's enough for Gerry? The answer is whatever keeps him injury-free and doing this shit he loves out of the gym. For 99.9 percent of us, how we lift is more important than how much we lift.

Safety First.

3 Risk vs. Reward

Living in a world where we are putting such high value on positivity and goal setting, we often go blind in pursuit of the reward. For some people this is called commitment; they have a deeper why, and it is a part of their very being. For others it is ignorance. They are neglecting to look at the potential risks associated in their egoic pursuits. The dry honesty is that the reward for hitting heavier lifts or consistently going hard in the gym doesn't always outweigh the risk.

"I am so glad I got that last PB on film," said Sally the childcare worker as she hobbled to her phone ignoring her impending lower-back injury. Anyway, my point once again isn't to not lift heavy. That's not what I am getting at. My point is to look at your programming, your exercise selection, and your intensity with an intelligent critical eye and ask if the reward outweighs the risk?

From there, let the client make a decision. Getting people strong is no good in the long term if they're also injured. Getting people fit is no good in the long term if they're simply avoiding other shit that they need to do in life.

Think past the 12-week transformation.

Think about the three-year e-mail you get from them thanking you for your patience and guidance.

It is so damn easy to get caught up in the moment and go after heavy lifts or stupidly hard workouts. I have been there. So many times! And in the long run, it is never worth it. Keep in mind this doesn't make everything black and white, yes or no. You as the coach may not know if the client/athlete should hit a heavier weight or not.

That's not your job.

Your job is to teach your client or athlete how to know their body.

To help them know whether to hit a heavier lift or whether it is their ego measuring against some arbitrary old goal that they have about being some number on a scale, as if happiness is only for those who weigh under 70 kg.

Does the risk of doing what you're about to do outweigh the reward?

It is the client's or athlete's job to know this. The coach is there to guide.

4 Teach; Don't Tell

In short, trainers tell and coaches teach. Trainers have good answers, and coaches have good questions. A good coach works with the client. They don't see them as someone who works for them and follows instruction. They meet them where they are at and work by their side to guide them to where they want to be. Unfortunately, for a lot of trainers (I was one of them), they will see clients as people who are to be told what to do, what to eat, and what to think. Although this may yield short-term results, it often sacrifices long-term progress.

Don't be a dictator with your clients. Work with them; get to know them. They are human beings with families, goals outside of the gym, emotions, and fears. Once you are able to build a real connection, you can make an epic difference to the long-term health of this individual. Achieving this creates long-term change not only in the individual but also the people closest to them. The goal is to get your client to not need you. Build them up; don't make them codependent because of your insecurities. Coach; don't just instruct. To teach is to learn twice. To tell is to order. People want to be lead and educated, and, overall, we want to be around an educated crowd as it encourages us to level up. When we only tell people what to do, we continue to build their dependency upon us, which in the short term allows them to stick around and pay us money to be personal trainers.

In the long term, people want to evolve and grow. Don't ever not teach your clients in fear of losing them. You have a better chance of referral when you educate them.

5 The Long Game

One of the common mistakes people (athletes, coaches, trainers, and clients) will make is to sacrifice long-term goals for short-term "wins." Without the long game top of mind we may find ourselves pursuing activities, numbers, or ego goals. For example, are you chasing a lift because it will make you perform well in the long term or are you trying to get a solid post for social media? Maybe it isn't as obvious as that. Maybe it is more subtle. Are you trying to prove something to someone rather than focusing on your long-term development?

By keeping the long game top of mind we are able to take a short-term loss. In fact, more often than not, those short-term losses set us up for the lessons we need to be able to have the long-term wins.

Short-term pleasure for long-term pain; short-term pain for long-term pleasure. More often than not, short-term pain has more to do with the ego than anything else.

Think macro, act micro. Those micromovements end up becoming large ones when they are added up over the years.

6 Cue One to Two

When I was a cowboy on the gym floor, I really wanted to dazzle people with all my knowledge. I wanted to be the guru and wanted to prove to people that I knew what I was talking about (even though I didn't really). Over time, I ended up gathering a decent amount of knowledge in training, nutrition, and mostly in the developmental space.

I then went on to vomit all the information I had on my clients still thinking that I would say the magic word to them and that this would win them over, and they would love me and everything would be okay with the world.

It was too much. Needless to say I was doing it for my reasons, not theirs, but I was also confusing them. Making them feel dumb. Overwhelmed. Therefore, I wasn't coaching, I was dictating. When I became aware that what I was doing was overwhelming and from the wrong place, I started to recognize that (like myself), we can only really focus on one or two things at any given time.

So I began to give one to two cues for the individual to focus on. I would watch the individual move and based on my assessment, I would consider which I thought was the most important factor for them to develop and would cue them on that rather than EVERYTHING they were doing "wrong." It is a simple and consumable approach to coaching and teaching, rather than drowning in deficiencies of what they weren't doing well.

These commandments are all about giving the right information to the right person at the right time. Because giving the right information to the right person at the wrong time is the wrong information.

7 Outcome Focused

One of the common mistakes trainers can get caught up in is giving clients a program, an exercise, or an approach that works for someone else. Often trainers will get caught up in the idea of "this is just how I coach."

That's lazy.

We as trainers or coaches should be committed to the outcome not the approach to getting to the outcome. If you are early on in your career, then I encourage you to get in front of as many clients and learn from as many coaches as you can. Fill your toolbox.

Have as many "activities" and "approaches" as possible and remember to be committed to the outcome for the client.

Where we make mistakes with this one is when we begin to be romantic about "the way"—the one way to do something, that that is the truth, and nothing else is true. My way is the right way, and it will most definitely get you your results.

And if it doesn't, you must have done something wrong. Let go of the one way to do it all. It's not just stalling your clients progress but also yours. Go out there and do all the research against your way. No matter how against it you are, try other things with an open mind. You haven't done all of the research and applied it to all the clients. It's not possible. Keep an open mind and remember that we are often "wrong" a lot before we are "right."

8 Student First

If you have committed to this industry, then you have also committed to lifelong learning. This rule alone means that you will always be in a position where you are not just the teacher but also the student. Even when teaching, there are things to be aware of that can help develop you as a coach and a trainer. At the core of every conversation, meeting, information transaction, and training session, you are the student because you can learn by observing different mechanics in individuals, different psychology, and responses let alone the feedback the individual is consciously saying and not saying.

If you are unable to learn the content or it is unavailable, then pay attention to the context. If you are at a presentation, how is the person speaking, standing, and giving their information? In each and every moment you are the student.

The other aspect of this commandment is that if you really want to make a mark on this industry and the people you come in contact with, then as a student, you study. You study every day. Whatever interests you the most, go all in on that. Get a mentor or a coach, or get two. Learn from them as much as you can no matter what your age and no matter how much you already know.

Always be hungrier for more knowledge.

All great leaders are great students.

9 Don't Fix

This feeds into (yet expands from) coaching commandment 3: Cue 1–2. We are taught early on to fix technique and, inadvertently, then fix clients. The issue with this is that it presupposes that someone is broken. This can create all types of issues that aren't even there in the first place. Good coaches don't fix people, they give them one to two things to focus on to improve. A good coach will be able to influence an individual to understand there is no right or wrong, that instead they are in a constant state of development.

We always have something to focus on. All of us. As a coach, it is your responsibility to bring that forward into your clients' or athletes' awareness for them to chip away at.

Often I have heard people who are early in the fitness journey come in and say to me, "Man! I have so much to work on." In response to which I inform them they have the same number of things to work on as I do.

One thing.

Focus on this one thing you are doing now. There is no finish line; we do this week in and week out. The big picture must be painted by focusing on the brush stroke you are currently creating with your paintbrush, not on the thousands that lie ahead of you.

Shift the conversation from fixing technique to improving movement or making it more efficient. If you are to see someone squat poorly, it is still a squat. It may just be inefficient. It doesn't make it wrong. They may have come a long way in improving that movement and are still just at stage 2 of 100 in improving it. Build this person; don't break them. So rather than fixing someone who isn't broken (you wouldn't do it to a child), give them a focus to help improve it. Don't look for right; look for better. There isn't an end point to any exercise, just an evolution.

10 Pace and Lead

One of the best ways to pace and lead an individual is to listen. And I mean truly listen. Listen with your whole body. What are you feeling? What is their breathing like? Is it shallow? Deep? Is it in the chest or the stomach? Are their eyes glazing over? Where are they looking? Is their voice strong or shaky? What are they not saying?

Truly great coaches don't just hear what their clients are saying, they are listening to everything. This is called sacred listening and is putting you in tune with the individual. When two people are in similar states, they feel more comfortable with each other and therefore more inclined to share and in return listen back.

To truly lead, you must meet the person where they are at. Meet firmness with compassion. Leadership with love. People don't hear that you care, they feel it. Once you are able to understand where the person is at both mentally and physically, then you are able to lead them from there.

This goes for all conversations where you have to sell something. Whether it be a membership or simply an information transaction to encourage that person to try something new in the gym that you know will benefit them in the long term.

Once you switch to true sacred listening, you can then truly lead.

11 Start Basic and Build

A mistake I have made too often in the past is creating some type of elaborate program, business plan or to-do list, and it became all too complicated and difficult. I never executed any of them.

I noticed the same thing in my clients and in my coaches. If we start complex, we often end up cutting things out. Now of course this can work, there are times I do create something complex and cut things out. With all these commandments, there will be the small minority of examples of the opposite being necessary.

When it comes to coaching, the issue surfaces when you remove stuff without framing it first. It can leave the individual feeling like they weren't good enough with the "norm" and need special consideration. It is far easier to start basic and build.

Same with your business. When starting out, it is common to have a lot of ideas, and they may be really good ideas. The issue is once again timing. You cannot do everything when you start. You may not have the infrastructure. So start basic and build. You have time.

12 Honey or Vinegar

American entrepreneur Gary Vaynerchuk talks about building a honey empire, and for the most part, I agree with him. What he is referring to is building people up with honey, with some love and nurturing.

This is a really different approach to that of the late Steve Jobs. In a coach-and-client relationship, start with honey. Don't get me wrong, tough love is important. That's the vinegar. And knowing when to apply it and to whom is crucial. More often than not, you build enough trust with 80 to 90 percent honey, which gives you leverage to be able to give that 10 to 20 percent vinegar, which is so critical for our development.

Coaching is the ability to know when to apply honey or vinegar and to whom. Sometimes those who need vinegar won't take it from you because you haven't earned their trust. This is often when you will hear something like, "I said that exact same thing to them, but they didn't listen to me!" Well maybe you hadn't earned their trust.

13 Rapport = Trust

One of the most common mistakes I see trainers make is that they try to build rapport because that is the thing you should do. The approach it from a tactical standpoint. True rapport isn't a tactic.

It's human interaction. It's visceral. You create rapport and look for sameness to understand the individual and to help meet them where they are at. You do it because you genuinely care. Not because it's in your mission statement.

There is a plethora of ways to build rapport, but the most important one is simply asking about how they are and things about them. This is so simple, and if you are able to do it from a place of both genuine interest and sincere caring, then you will build rapport. It's no mistake that the word "trust" is so similar to the word "truth." If something in your approach is false, it will be felt, and rapport will be broken, which, in turn, means trust will also be lost. By listening, asking questions, pacing, giving a focus, starting basic, and giving one to two cues you can help build rapport.

Couple any of these with unconditional patience, and you will most likely build long-term trust.

You can break rapport by correcting, fixing, or telling, which in the long run will make building trust that much more challenging.

Before we impart our wisdom, we must first build rapport.

14 Mature and Then Grow

One of the biggest lessons I learned was to not grow too quickly. We keep what we earn. Often people will take for granted what came easy. I have seen a lot of people lose what they gained fast. So no matter what you're doing, don't worry about exploding onto the scene, be patient. Build your personal empire (read mission, life, house, business, not for profit) with bricks not sticks.

Now, apply this commandment to coaching rather than just your career; short-term strength gains will often yield injuries that patience and slow incremental improvements can avoid almost every time.

Whether it be in business, training, the mind, or any aspect in life in which we want to grow, we must first mature.

It could be argued that all maturity is growth but not all growth is maturity.

15 Behavioral Adaptability

The overarching commandment the one that glues all the others together is behavioral adaptability.

If we stay firm in who we are, understand ourselves, and adapt our behavior, our communication, and physiology based on the people we interact with every day, then we can truly begin to unravel our potential and make a positive impact on a larger scale.

All the above commandments heavily depend on the flexibility we apply to each and every individual. Once again, this depends greatly on how well we understand ourselves.

I urge you to constantly be the student, learn all areas of human performance and human potential, always approach every person you meet as a potential teacher and as if they know something you don't, because they do.

The overarching principle for all of us is conscious behavioral adaptability while acting in accordance to our true selves.

*   *   *

At the end of the day, we want to be able to celebrate what our body can do, not punish it because of the way we eat or think. Ideally our training should help fuel our lives outside of the gym and become a lifelong learning process along the way. There are so many different ways to train and different motivations to train. My offer is to be patient with yourself and find a way to celebrate movement that enhances your life outside of just movement. My other offer is for you to keep challenging yourself both physically and mentally.

Keep making memories.

PART III

The
FOOD

Mouth and Nutrition

Over the following pages, I will have Nick Shaw from Renaissance Periodization (a.k.a. "RP"; https://renaissanceperiodization.com/) assisting me by providing the most up-to-date, relatable, and evidence-based information. Nick Shaw and his highly qualified team at RP have helped hundreds of thousands of people all over the world through their nutrition templates, online lectures, and social media platforms. At the time of this writing, their team boasts twenty PhDs, seven registered dieticians, plus professors, research scientists, doctors, world champions, and collegiate-level sports coaches.

Although some of our information may be communicated differently as we both have different backgrounds and come at nutrition from slightly different angles, it is the integration of all our information and knowledge that will yield you the most success as you develop your nutritional habits and education.

Nick Shaw and RP have an extensive online educational platform called RP+ that can keep you busy for years to come with its depth and science-backed research/lectures.

Moving forward we will be referring to a few different models. The first of these models is the HIQ Mouth Map. We will be covering the three different levels of nutrition, so you are in a position to best identify where you are at and where you need to be based on your goals and desired outcomes.

Those three levels are the following:

- Simple
- Sustainable
- Specific

For long-term development in all areas of the HIQ Map, it is about moving through the stages as necessary.

Everybody's end game will be different, and it is not about needing to get to *specific* but rather about finding a balance that will suit them in their life whether that be to keep things *simple*, maintain something *sustainable* for their life, or to move toward a more specific outcome or goal from time to time.

The key thing to remember is that it is about transcending and including the different stages of nutrition.

Once you have made things simple and you have that covered, start to move to a long-term sustainable approach that includes the goals you have with your life. "Sustainable" doesn't just apply to sustainable eating but also sustainable for the planet, sustainable for your life goals, and sustainable for your relationships.

The specific end of the nutrition stage is often seen as short-term peaks of discipline for a specific goal. The way it works is that if someone was to jump straight here without doing the work and education at the lower levels, then when the goal is either over or no longer desirable, the person will return to the baseline level of their HIQ. Hence the yo-yo cycle.

By doing the time and learning the lessons in the simple and sustainable levels, someone who peaks into specific will then return to a long-term sustainable approach rather than dropping back to simple or below. Hence, it reduces the yo-yo and the guilt that is so often associated with eating particular foods.

"We don't rise to the occasion; we fall to our training."

It is easy to overcomplicate things when it comes to nutrition. There are plenty of different diets and different ways to address nutrition and for the most part, they all "work."

More often than not the question is more about what is sustainable for the lifestyle you want and how much different is that to where you are currently at?

A couple of main things we want to consider when it comes to nutrition are the following:

1. Is this a short-term or long-term goal?

2. Do I have what is considered a "healthy" relationship with food?

Often people can get caught up attempting to create a long-term change in their life by short-term discipline. What is recommended is to think macro and act micro. That is to think long term while making short-term decisions that lead to the success of a long-term vision.

Neither short-term goals nor long-term goals are better than the other. It is the integration of both that allows for long-term change and success.

A long-term goal without short-term goals (think of them as checkpoints) is often too long for people to stay the path. There are also so many changes that can occur in one's life and in the world around one to stay true to a long-term goal without revising, realigning, and editing course as necessary. Short-term checkpoints that act as short-term goals allow us to not only feel motivated by the action we have created but also to reassess where we are at and what changes if any we need to make to edit the course.

A short-term goal (or a string of short-term goals) without a long-term goal or vision can lead someone to become sporadic and ungrounded. They can feel successful as they tick things off their bucket list but unfulfilled in a way that only real long-term success and purpose can fuel. This person often lacks long-term direction and the patience to build a foundation. Interestingly, what they are searching for in their short-term success can be found in long-term purpose.

A long-term vision that is peppered with short-term goals allows for long-term success and fulfillment.

Hence the question "What happens on day 31 of the 30-day challenge?" is absolutely crucial.

I often communicate to clients starting out that I simply am not interested in a 12-week before and after nearly as much as I am interested in an e-mail in three years saying thank you: Thank you for your guidance as I was able to ski with my family for a week on holidays without any knee pain or watching from the sidelines. Thank you for giving me the opportunity to take responsibility for my health; my kids have started to ask more questions about food and where it comes from. Thank you for supporting me; I was able to pass the fitness test required of special forces.

Whatever the thank you is, it was more than 12 weeks before and after.

Twelve-week challenges or before and afters are valid in their own right; the issues, however, come with how often we need to keep challenging ourselves to be "healthy." It simply isn't healthy to keep restricting ourselves so that we don't be "naughty" and flog ourselves at the gym to get some sort of short-term result time after time. It is mentally, emotionally, and physically damaging. It is literally the food and training equivalent of binge drinking on weekends or once a month.

Sometimes 12-week challenges can be the start of momentum to a long-term healthier version of ourselves. So 12-week challenges aren't out. Binging on challenges over years to meet a number on a scale is out.

For many reasons.

One of the reasons is that there is a generation below us watching us. Naughty foods, punishing ourselves at the gym, and basing happiness on external factors are being observed and copied by those who look up to us. When we rid ourselves of these out-of-date practices, we rid the next generation of them too.

If we really want to make long-term change, then we must think past just ourselves and our lifetime.

When someone comes into my gym and tells me they want to lose weight, they aren't just saying they want a lower number on the scales. They want what they think that number will represent. There is a small opportunity to help this person change the course of their future grandchildren, grandchildren who may not even be born yet.

So the issue with the 12-week transformations isn't the results. It is the fact that it often stops at the results and we rarely ever progress. In most cases, they regress. It is literally just a long-term version of a yo-yo.

Another of the main reasons is that people end up yo-yoing as they take too large a jump from their current lifestyle and belief structure to their ideal lifestyle and belief structure. Or they don't even address their belief structure at all and think it is just what they are eating or how they aren't exercising. They neglect to realize that we build our habits because of our thoughts. We can change the habits, but the thoughts must evolve and change too.

Another issue can be that it isn't their ideal lifestyle that they shift to. It was simply the best-marketed diet at the time that gave them hope that "this time it will work." In other words, people will pursue a marketed "lifestyle" that appears happier or sexier or more appealing than their own. They are pursuing an image of health rather than learning what health is to them, which quite frankly isn't healthy.

One problematic phrase that I have heard countless times over the past 15 years is "I/we don't eat bad. We will only have takeout once a week, if that" or something to that effect. To clarify, "takeout" or "takeaway" means food cooked at a fast-food restaurant or similar outlet.

The issue with this isn't around the takeout. It is thinking that everything but takeout is "healthy."

One of the most important things that we need to do is to continually be able to define what health is to ourselves. I say continually because what demands you have in your life and what needs your body and mind will have will change over the years. We have an opportunity to continually be in touch with our mind-body connection and to truly be in touch with ourselves. True development of HIQ is a process, an unravelling of ourselves over years, not a static screenshot of a moment in our life, a doctor's script or a PR or a diet plan. It is continually being connected within ourselves for life.

Another important question to ask is, how long can I realistically maintain this as a standard?

The key word here is "sustainability." Not everything we do with food has to be sustainable all the time. Which, ironically enough, makes it sustainable. Short-term goals can often call for more disciplined actions toward food and exercise. The key difference is knowing that it is short term. Practically speaking we can peak into a stricter eating plan and training regime. We just have to be clear and honest with ourselves if this is going to be something that we can maintain and if so, how long can we maintain it?

Another way to pose the question is how long do I need to hold this standard before my goal is achieved? Then, do I have the ability to maintain that plan for that period of time?

Sometimes the answer is "No, I don't," and that is completely okay. Self-honesty is the most crucial form of honesty there is.

If the answer was to be "No I don't," then the next question is "What can I do that I would do that will allow me to work toward my goal today?"

Our ability to ask ourselves powerful and compelling questions is directly correlated with our successful pursuit of a worthy goal. I believe it was Tony Robbins who said that the quality of our life is dependent on the quality of our questions. We already have all the answers, it is the questions we seek.

"It is better to have questions you cannot answer than answers you cannot question." – Anon.

The same principle of making short-term behavioral change based on goals also applies to relaxing an eating plan. For example, over the Christmas holiday period somebody may be more likely to relax their nutrition plan more and enjoy a few more alcoholic drinks than usual. During this time they don't identify as being naughty, binging, or being lazy. They are simply adjusting to their own measurement of what health is for them and are able to make decisions based on what is required of them in the moment.

Come January 1 they won't need to go to the gym and bash out all the bad things they ate, and they won't feel the urge to restrict themselves to some grapefruit juice diet. They will simply return to my baseline.

Now if they had a specific goal that they wanted to reach or achieve in January, then they would simply readdress their short-term behaviors based off this goal knowing that they will return to their baseline after the goal has been achieved.

Nutrition Grading

So we can get a good grounding of where we are at, where we want to go, and how to get there; let's use the example of grading someone on a similar grading scale that schools use to grade students except, we are using it for nutrition.

This grading system allows us to identify where people are at on the HIQ Map and, more importantly, where they need to be to align with their goals.

The grading system operates on a scale from A (highest) through to E (lowest).

Each grade will also have a + (plus) and a – (minus). Because this model is a dynamic model, the +/– are there to signify when people are either shifting, growing/emerging, or regressing through the grades.

These grades can also be referred to as either stages or levels. Unlike school, where it may be perceived that it is always best to get an A grade in everything, we recommend that the grade that best correlates to your goals that you have in life is the best grade for you. Different stages of life call for different demands and stresses and therefore different grades. We are all unfolding at different times and stages; there is no one right way to do so.

Your ideal grade based on your goals could be either be a C or a B grading or maybe it is an A. It greatly depends on what is needed of you during that time in your life.

The gradings are both subjective and objective. They are subjective in the way that they can be complex and fluid, and what is often the most important factor in which grade someone is dependent upon their intention and context. For example, someone may be snacking on foods that aren't in their usual plan because they feel like it on that day. They will have absolutely no guilt associated with eating the snack and may genuinely just want to enjoy the experience of having that individual snack. Another person may be doing the exact same thing; however, they may be coming from a place of pleasing cravings and caving into the food, therefore handing their power over and relinquishing their ability to choose. A lot of the time, you can see these two types of people at a party, and you may struggle to tell the difference between the two. Same behaviors, different intent, different stages.

Each grade will have a corresponding stage on the HIQ Map. This allows us to not only define our grade in nutrition, but to understand where our stage is on the map.

There are many factors that go into the type of education required to move through each grade. I have made a brief breakdown about the common type of education that goes into developing a person's ability to reach each grade.

Everyone has a bandwidth on the grading scale. What this means is that we will have access to some higher levels and some lower levels. This also means that we have a gravitational grade that we spend most of our time at. We refer to this as our baseline. This is where you spend most of your time and where you are most comfortable every day. As we develop, our grade develops, and with it, our baseline.

The lower levels in the bandwidth are available to us when we are under unusual levels of stress. We refer to this as the "stress anchor." What this means is that we are likely to drop down the grading a little bit when we have more urgent priorities. Some examples could be moving house, changing jobs, change in relationship status. To have access to our stress anchor allows us to pull back some pressure, reassess, regroup, and move forward again. Our stress anchor is not a bad place. It is necessary for us to have access to and have flexibility with it. If we don't have healthy access to this stress anchor level, we can often fall apart trying to hold it all together and then we are more susceptible to a diet crash.

We also have access to a peak state. A peak state is where we have bouts of what is perceived to be increased amounts of discipline. This is when we are able to reach a higher grading for small bouts of time. We usually do this when we are secure and stable. Over time and with continual self-work, education, and experience our peak state can become our baseline stage thus usually gaining access to a higher peak nutritional state.

The beautiful thing about this grading model is that as you move from E to A, you transcend and include the lower grades of development. This means that when you emerge into a higher level, you take all the experience and learnings from the lower grades with you. At the higher grades, you see the utility of the lower grades. It is a normal part of the transition.

Remember: this grading scale is a guide. It allows us to gauge where our current baseline is and recognize where we are most likely to gravitate to 80 to 90 percent of the time.

Allow me to preframe that a grade can simply be an A– or a B+ depending on where the person mainly gravitates to with their nutrition. For example, someone who does most of the B grade standards but likely leans into C grade standards from time to time would be considered a B– grade student.

Everybody's bandwidth along the grading will vary and is neither wrong nor right. It just is where it is at. Our baseline is heavily influenced by a number of factors:

- Nutritional education
- Belief structures
- Self-image/identity
- Social groups
- Environment
- Parenting
- Goals (past and present)
- Relationships

Considering that these are just some of the factors involved when aiming to improve our baseline and consequently increasing our HIQ, the truth is that it will take time and work. The good news is that the time will pass anyway, whether you do it or not.

Being told what to eat rather than learning what we need to eat, for what goal and why, makes for a big difference when spread out over years. One is often associated with a lower grading and lower level of responsibility and the other with a higher grading and a healthy level of responsibility. What is interesting though is that seeking assistance and being told what to eat is a step above unconsciously consuming and avoiding nutritional education, which is apparent in the lower grades. Therefore, seeking assistance and guidance is a necessary part of the development up through the grades.

We have to move through all stages to get from E right through to A. You cannot skip any stages or you risk a regression to below that stage.

When we are young, we are simply told what to eat and eat what our parents eat. There are some little rebels and mismatchers out there who went against their parents' word, but for the most part, if we didn't eat what was put in front of us, we didn't eat. This is simply associated with a lower level of grading because it is what is necessary at that stage of development. As we begin to get older, we start to have different interests and goals (or maybe concerns) and will start to seek guidance and education in the area of nutrition. This is why it is important to understand that we are just at wherever we are at.

What's important is to find out what level best supports our life's goals and then learn what we need to do to move toward that level.

It should also be stressed that the goal for everyone isn't to be an A grade student unless that is the level that best supports your goals and life. Aiming for that level can actually become detrimental to many facets of our life. The goal is to be able to have a baseline HIQ level that supports your goals and life-long term while having access to the levels on either of your baseline.

I refer to the people associated with each grade as a "student," which is in reference to the lifelong learning we have with nutrition and living.

Here are a few questions that may help you as you read through the grades:

What grade best describes how I spend most of my day/week?

What behaviors and thoughts do I have access to when I have a worthy goal?

What behaviors best describe me in times of stress or unease?

The answers to these questions should help you gauge where your baseline is, your peak nutritional state, and your stress anchor.

Below are the student grades starting at E although way through to A. I have also aligned these grades up with the stages on the HIQ Map so that you can better grasp where nutritional behaviors, thoughts and education sit.

You will notice that there are some grades that are not positioned on the HIQ Map. That is because these grades sit below the action and implementation stage of wanting to improve. Because of this, they are the pre-stages of development on the HIQ Map.

A Grade Student: They follow a nutrition plan to the exact amounts to be eaten and exact eating times. They have "cheat" meals sparingly and find it easy to live their lifestyle in a way that coincides with their food plans. They no longer diet; this is just what they have conditioned themselves to eat. They see food as a source of energy and what it allows them to experience in their life. That is, they enjoy food but take more fulfillment from what it allows them to do and the freedom it has enriched their lives with than the feeling of enjoyment from eating the food.

Education: A grade students have invested years into their lives learning about all the facets of nutrition. They have learned about multiple types of "diets" and developed a healthy overarching group of principles that help direct their nutritional decisions. They take total responsibility for their health as they no longer see separation between mind and body but rather an integration of health and fitness through a mind-body connection.

They start to see the extreme ways in their old nutrition patterns and have found a healthy balance for themselves and their lives. They can switch on the ability to be more precise and specific with their nutrition for a specific goal as well as the ability to dial it back to a healthy level post goal.

A+ Grade: The only way to be able to obtain this level is through conscious experience and persistence. It often takes years to get to a place where you can pivot your diet and have full control of what serves you in every moment as opposed to being a puppet to a program with no deep connection to the long-term result. People in this range can be anyone from an elite level bodybuilder right through to your neighbor next door. Not everyone in this stage will look the same although they have gone through all the educational learnings and personal discoveries along the way to becoming the healthiest versions of themselves inside and out.

A− Grade: The shift from B+ to A− can often be the biggest jump out of all of the stages. After acquiring all of the knowledge and science required to become so well versed and intelligent, they start to move into seeing other perceptions of what is healthy outside of calories in versus calories out.

They move from seeing health as a perfect diet and training regime to flexibility based on their life conditions and stages of development. They no longer are controlled by their regime but rather have control of their regime. What makes this jump so challenging for many is that they have invested so much time, money, and energy in learning the exact right plan and program for them only to realize there is still something missing, that happiness isn't a diet plan or training program. That there is more to it. If discipline equals freedom, they then begin to learn that too much self-discipline is tyranny upon oneself.

It often takes time and sometimes a bit of resisting, but after much personal and internal debate, they begin to relax more while still making value-driven decisions.

HIQ MAP: A graders can move through the different stages of the map at will. They are not tied down to a specific (or the specific) level as they have transcended and included all levels of the HIQ Map. They are also patient with other people at other stages and respect the journey. They are usually genuinely humble and happy to offer advice and also happy to stay silent. They have a larger picture of what health is and know that everyone is simply unfolding at their own rate. They understand the importance of all levels, and their key attribute in relation to the map is their flexibility to move through the levels with ease and without anyone knowing.

B Grade Student: They follow a nutrition plan to pretty much the exact amounts and have a small window either side of their exact eating times. They embrace "cheat" meals and will meal prep for the week ahead. They make conscious decisions with their nutrition even when they are out although they will likely have a massive intake once or twice a month. They can often be black-plus-white thinkers and although this can help them get amazing physiques, it can impact their true, pure enjoyment in life.

Education: They have started to take more personal responsibility for their own health and knowledge of what food is and isn't. They are likely to follow more science-based information and principles when it comes to nutrition. They can sometimes be caught in the all or nothing phase with nutrition, which will more often still end in the "nothing" space from time to time. In this grade, people still cover up old tendencies and coping mechanisms with food or exercise. This is what keeps them from being an A student. They are yet to integrate a healthy frame of mind into their extensive nutrition knowledge.

B+ Grade: This is the emerging grade for B grade students, where they really start to lean into the flexibility of what is required of them long term. They are often sick of the do-or-die attitude and start to move into experiencing life with more love for the moment while keeping long-term goals and progression in mind. They shift from always saying no to things that they love, that they used to call "sacrifices" to realize that they were simply only sacrificing parts of their lives for an image or to prove someone wrong or something similar.

B– Grade: Somebody moves into this grade once they really start to delve deeper into their education and understanding of how food impacts their body. Usually, they will start with one type of diet research, for example, something that has worked for them in the past: Keto, Paleo, Vegetarianism, and so on.

The B– grade is often where real research begins. This stage is important to develop because even though at this stage the person is often a-one trick pony, they begin to value education and have started to open their mind to the power food has over our body and our mind. In turn, this is the first real stage of personal responsibility because they aren't just taking responsibility for what goes in their body from a food perspective but also what goes into their mind from a knowledge perspective.

HIQ MAP: B+ Grade students can be really starting to emerge with their nutrition flexibility, whereas B– students are becoming more and more rigid with how specific they need to be. Hence their shift into the top level of the map, specific. Traditionally B grade students will be very concise and regimented with their specific level and haven't yet gained full access to the flexibility and the power of choice that A grade students have access to. Although they have transcended the lower levels of simple and sustainable, they are yet to integrate them and include them. Over time, if the B student continues to develop, they will begin to integrate and shift from a B+ through to an A– and begin to have a nutrition plan rather than being had by it.

C Grade Student: Overall this student lives a pretty healthy life when it comes to nutrition. For the most part they eat four to five meals a day of decent, semi-nutritious food. They are more relaxed when it comes to serving amounts. They will grab food on the go from time to time, and even though they do, they can't help but feel a little bit guilty about it.

This is where most of the population will sit, give or take a –/+. They are conscious of what is most likely a better option without being educated in depth with how the food they consume impacts their energy, health, mental health, and long-term physical health.

Education: Most of their education comes from a small bit of research online, mainstream marketing, or following some influencers and their recommendations. (HINT: Influencers are marketers.) They still have a lot of old educational beliefs passed on by caregivers. You hear it in their language when they say something like "everything in moderation."

What is wrong with moderation you may ask? Well nothing, besides *who* defines it. Moderation was probably good advice a couple of generations ago when moderation was in reference to the food you had access to locally and was home grown. Moderation today includes Uber eats, multiple fast-food outlets, and frozen food delivered from all around the world. In 100 years, moderation again will look very different. One person's moderation may be up there with a C or B grade. Another person may be closer to a D or E grading.

C+ Grade: We start to see this come online for someone when they are curious about learning the how and why behind the what of nutrition. They may not be researching or furthering their education yet but are growingly curious about what they should eat. This first develops in the mind and then they likely either start doing some google searches or ask people in their trusted circle. As a gym coach, I am very mindful when someone first presents a nutrition question as it may be this grade emerging and coming online for them. If that is the case, I can point them in the direction to learn more. Where coaches can sometimes go wrong is in simply just giving them a diet plan. Sometimes they ask for a plan, but it isn't always what they want. It can even stall their development for weeks or even months. Maybe even years. This isn't to say that the plan isn't important for this stage of development, it is. But the plan with some questions or further research can start to open doors for people to really start taking responsibility for their health and nutrition. It is crucial at this level to keep it simple. Do not overcomplicate things and start basic and then build more and more into the learning and food plan.

C– Grade: These individuals have started to make "better" choices with their food with the knowledge that they currently have. They will start purchasing "fat-free" foods or low-sugar foods, and foods with a higher health rating, even if it is cereal. They are beginning to become health conscious but lack the drive or even awareness to start researching and educating themselves about food and nutrition. This is often where some health kick-starts for some people as they may want to do something by themselves because they are too embarrassed to ask for help or maybe they are still slightly in denial that they may need it or at least benefit from it. People at this stage may start asking but can be proud in their response as they -ay not want to look stupid. Once they start researching (usually in private so they have some type of information to bring to the table when asking for help), they start to move into the C grade.

HIQ MAP: We start to see the simple stage of development come on strongest in the C+ grade of development. Although it starts to show its face at earlier levels such as C and possibly even C–, we don't see it fully come on until the person starts taking ownership of their health, nutrition, and education. In the earlier stages of

C and C–, we see it in the way people may take care of their kids and keep things simple or keep dinners simple; however, it really doesn't begin to appear until they start taking responsibility for their own health. During this period, there may be a desire to jump ahead and either be told what to do or they attempt to get too specific. Because the individuals haven't spent a lot of time developing the basics ("simple" stage), getting too specific too soon can be detrimental. It can cause the person to take on too much change, which can be an overload of stress, and being successful with the changes made in training and nutrition can be too much for the belief structure that person holds and therefore they simply drop everything. Start basic with people here and build, not in a complex way, and then cut things out. Giving people at this level A or B grade information and nutritional plans can be likened to giving a music student who is starting out a sheet of one of Beethoven's symphony to learn. Start basic.

D Grade Students: These students are aware they don't eat well but may not be aware just how bad they are eating and, frankly, often just don't care (yet). They likely were never taught about food, and their parents either ignored the conversation altogether because of their lack of awareness and knowledge about food or they simply didn't think it was important. Food is food right? Usually deep down these individuals know what they are eating is bad for long-term health, but they think they can "get away with it" for years or maybe even the rest of their lives. It is often not until they have a health scare that they start to think that maybe they need to do something about their diet. And then, depending on their response, they will determine whether or not they climb the grading, stay where they are, or become apathetic and nihilistic and drop down the grading. People here don't see health as something they really have much control over. They suggest that most of their issues are hereditary and unlikely be impacted positively by anything other than pharmaceutical drugs. They can become a victim to their health issues if they regress or even if they stay at this grade.

At a young age, children will be in this area as they start to identify what foods are dinner foods, snack foods, and breakfast foods. This period in a child's development can be a heavily impactful time if parents are not mindful and thoughtful when presenting food options and talking about food. I personally recall a time where my dear mother brought my lunch to school. We lived in a small country town at the time, and my mother and her partner managed the local hotel. She would grab a beef and gravy roll from the kitchen in the hotel and then also a pink donut and a carbonated energy drink for me. I was 11. I was told I would burn it off. That type of thinking (and eating) can end up causing some long-term issues as an adult if the child doesn't develop through the levels of grades and learns to take responsibility for its health and eating.

Education: Education at this grade is often the information that was passed down to people by their caregivers and what is marketed on either TV or the Internet. Without the urge to pursue further personal education, people here simply continue repeating sentiments from long ago that have lived on from generation to generation. It is not often their health that is hereditary as much as it is their family values and perception of the world.

D+ Grade: At this level people want to change; they just don't know how, and it may initially appear all too hard. They aren't quite ready yet to take responsibility for their health and food choices. They live habitually and defined by eating patterns from when they were younger and, as mentioned, although they want to change, there is still more pain associated with change than not to changing. At this level, a helpful friend or a caring coach can be a big help to get the person over the line. Often this person first needs to do some form of exercise before they will start to make nutritional changes. The endorphins and feeling of accomplishment they get from walking the block, going to the gym, or seeing the scales drop a little bit can often motivate them into wanting to learn more. Giving this person a low barrier opportunity that withholds judgment is one of the best ways for them to step into their journey of education and nutrition. Often the transition from here to the B grade average can take years. But, as mentioned before, that time will pass anyway.

D– Grade: People at this level not only don't want to change but also don't see the point in changing. They are often completely lack responsibility, irrational when it comes to food, and often have a self-image that is committed to staying this way. In fact, if they were to lose weight and become healthier, they wouldn't know who they would be anymore because this is all they have ever known. Their father was like that and their father's father and their fathers, fathers, father. Often these persons' loved ones can see what poor nutrition is doing to them and to their family; however, this person wants to be left alone in their habits and vices (not that they see them as vices). They may even start shutting people off who annoy them with them wanting to change.

HIQ MAP: The D grade is the pre-stage of simple on the HIQ Map. They are usually not ready to take ownership and make changes; however, late stage D+ start to gain the desire to learn. This is really the first stage of consideration on the HIQ Map. I call it consideration because it is usually only a desire for change and not actual change, nor any actual action taken. There is usually no action until the person moves into the C grade stage; however, desire builds in this stage, and that is important as desire must first occur before one can move into the C grade stage of action. Therefore the D grade is as necessary as any other to move through in order to build long-term health as it builds the initial desire to get better. Once the desire to improve outweighs the pain of staying wherever they currently are, the person will begin to move into the C gradings.

E Grade Student: Individuals at this level are oblivious to the power food has for their health, happiness, and freedom of life. They aren't aware of how the food we eat impacts the environment and are often around other individuals in this level and D grade levels. They see people who make healthier food choices as "those people" or "healthy people" as they don't identify as a healthy person or care to learn what the benefits are. At higher levels, we learn that there aren't healthy or unhealthy people. There are just people; some make healthy choices, and some make less healthy choices. At higher stages, they see it as a continuum rather than a black-and-white identity of this or that.

Individuals at this level are unaware of how much power advertising, marketing, and food in general has over them. They are often consumers and think that what they do is "normal."

HIQ MAP: People in the E grade stage of development have usually just accepted that what they are like now is how they always have been and always will be. "There are those people and then there is us." This stage doesn't register on the HIQ Map as they are completely unaware of either the importance of nutrition or its impact on them and the world.

As you can see, not everyone needs to be an A student. Any level at any time can serve you depending on your life conditions and what is required of you at that moment. If you normally gravitate toward a B+, and someone close to you, let's say your spouse is omitted to the emergency room all of a sudden, chances are your nutrition is no longer as important to you as it once was. Hence the ability to drop down the grading to something that will be more suitable for you in that moment.

This is the power of flexibility, self-awareness, and self-honesty. This is the power of moving from an all or nothing attitude that has power over you to a grading scale that you have power over.

What is the F grading I hear you ask? It is where you aren't eating at all. It may often lead to death. Therefore, it is a failed mark. My humble advice: try not to spend too much time here.

Nutrition 101—Keep It Simple

It's Just Food.

One of the most powerful distinctions we can make about what we eat is the distinction between food and not food. Not food can also be referred to as CRAP: carbonated, refined, artificial, and processed.

One of the issues that have come up in the last 100 years is this idea of "healthy food." Most food is only referred to as healthy because it has unhealthy food to compare to. Unfortunately, the other food isn't called unhealthy food often. It is called food.

At some point, we changed from calling what we considered as food, by added a little word at the start, to call it "healthy food."

This may not seem like a bad thing and, to be fair, it wasn't a BAD thing. But the issues that it can cause are based upon people's identities. For example, there are certain foods we eat when we go on a "health kick" and change from the foods we eat normally.

If it is healthy food and I don't identify as a healthy person, then I am going to have some big trouble transitioning to the healthy food from "normal" food.

The reality is that it is just food. It grew from the ground or it had a mum (mom, for you Americans). It isn't healthy food; it's not for healthy people. It is food, it is what humans eat. The healthy part is mainly there for marketing purposes, just like there is a health food isle at your local supermarket. And surprise, surprise, it isn't the grocery section. In fact, it is usually all man made.

If that aisle is the health food aisle, what kind of food is in all the other aisles?

There are a few distinctions that should be heavily considered when looking at food and long-term health. The way that we view and communicate about food can often say a lot about our relationship with food. For example, most people will have a negative connotation or emotional response toward the word "diet." In my experience, terms that often come up for (most) people are words like:

- Short term
- Restriction
- Fad
- Hard
- Weight loss

The greater part of society has a negative emotional response to the very thing that we are trying to fix.

This doesn't mean every single human will see this word in this way; it means a lot of us grew seeing our parents going on a "diet" and being absolutely miserable. Who would want to grow up and be like that?

Unfortunately, a lot of us did whether we wanted to or not because that's all we knew. It is what we saw adults to be like, so a large majority of us modelled ourselves on them.

One thing we can do about this is to remove the negative emotional stigma attached to the word diet; the other thing would be to use a different word that may be a more fitting description.

By simply referring to what we eat as nutrition rather than diet we can change the whole emotional response we have to food. This doesn't mean that this little shift will single handedly make someone healthier. It is only one component of a bigger solution. There is no one solution; it is a combination of small changes that make the overall shift.

The other big player in the negative emotional response team when it comes to "dieting" is the trusty old cheat meal.

Growing up (hopefully), most of us were taught that cheating was inherently bad, that it is morally wrong, and if we get caught cheating, we will be punished. So let's get our emotionally traumatic idea of going on a diet and throw in some cheat meals to make sure we have a good excuse to punish ourselves at the gym for being naughty.

This type of thinking is causing the problem; it is promising to fix.

Don't cheat on a diet; don't reward yourself with food (you're not a dog), and snack foods aren't treats (yep, still not a dog). The goal here is being able to see food as food, not as an emotional response that controls your cravings and self-esteem.

If you are following a nutritional plan and you have a meal that would be traditionally be called a cheat meal, then why don't you shift to calling it something more fitting like a "relaxed meal"?

Relax. Don't count the calories on this one. There is no judgment besides the one you pass on yourself. You aren't cheating; it is part of the plan.

Just enjoy your food for what it is: food.

To master the simple stage on the HIQ Map, we have to first learn to identify what foods we eat that are considered protein sources, carbohydrate sources, and fat sources. Protein, carbs, and fats (P/C/F) are known as macronutrients. To some people this is common knowledge; however, it should not be overlooked because at some point we didn't know what protein, carb, or fat was.

So before we go handing out diets to follow, we must learn the simple aspects to nutrition to be able to build a base for everything else to be built on top of it.

One of the easiest ways to understand the difference between proteins and carbs is that protein moves around; carbohydrates grow in the ground. Of course, this is a nice anecdotal way to identify protein and carbs; there are plenty of protein sources that may also grow in the ground, especially if you are wanting to follow either a vegetarian or a vegan-style nutrition plan.

The Five Simple Steps

This is my five-step process to starting out with learning how to take control of your eating and nutrition planning. Of course, it is easier to just hand over a plan and say follow this, and as explained earlier in this book you are likely to get shorter term results from this. Instead I recommend starting slow and simple and building from there so that we can take the lessons from week to week.

Each step can take different amounts of time. It may take one or two weeks to understand a particular step and meet the criteria of that step, or it may take a couple of hours on a Sunday afternoon. If it takes longer, then it takes longer. There is no right amount of time per step.

For some people, these steps will be great to build a foundation; for others they may be too simple. If you already have these steps covered and meet the KPI in each step then by all means move onto the sustainable stage. If not, then follow these simple steps to increase your HIQ.

Step 1
Write everything down

For the most part, I am against a diet diary. The diet diary falls short as a long-term solution because although the idea is to write down and become conscious of what you are consuming and eating, it often reinstalls guilt, negative emotions to foods, and I have even seen people lie about them so that they "don't get in trouble."

A diet diary is a reactive way to address our nutritional education. All this aside, the diet diary is how we start the five steps. We use it as an opportunity to benchmark where our nutrition is currently at so we have a starting point. The more descriptive, the better. There is no shame in whatever we write down; it just is what it is. Honesty is so important here as a lack of integrity will likely show its face later on and jeopardize all the work that has gone into it. Be clear and as precise in this step.

KPIs

Write down everything you eat for one week in as much detail as possible. Include timings of meals where possible.

That's it! Step 1 done! Simple, isn't it?

Step 2
Fill in the gaps

After writing out one week's worth of food, take a look at your diary, and start recognizing the days where you ate less than three meals. Aim to fill in these days with somewhere between four to five meals. The goal of this step is to start getting used to eating regularly and eating enough.

This is the first stage of moving from recording to planning. There is a massive difference between a diet diary and a nutrition plan. One is reactive, that is, to re-action behaviors of the past. The other is proactive, meaning to choose new behaviors that best serve a worthy goal.

If you are already eating four to five meals a day then great! Give yourself a pat on the back and move onto step 3.

KPIs

Ensure you have four to five meals per day. They can vary in size; the important thing in the beginning is that you are making sure you are in the habit of being conscious of your eating and eating regularly.

Step 3
Identify P/C/F

Using your diary from the previous two steps, start to identify the P/C/F sources in each meal. **That is, using the foods guide provided**, identify which foods in each of your meals are your protein source, carbohydrate source, and fat source.

Don't worry if some meals don't have all three. In this step we just want to start the learning process of which meals have what. You can do this by using the previous one to two weeks of diary recording before starting the next week.

KPIs

Start to identify in each meal what is your protein, carbohydrate, and fat source. If needed, use the guide provided to identify what foods are P, C, and F sources. Mark down a P, C, or F next to the meal/food item.

Step 4
Add PCF where missing

Now that we have recorded our baseline for our eating habits, consistently eat at least four meals a day and identified what macronutrients are in each meal, we are going to add in any macronutrients that may be missing from each meal. For example, if you have a meal that only has a carb and a fat source, add in a protein. If you have a meal that is just a protein and fat source, add in a carbohydrate.

We are not concerning ourselves about serving sizes and types of macronutrients yet. We just want to get into the habit of recognizing what a PCF is and eating consistently.

KPIs

Over the next week as you plan your nutrition, identify where you are not meeting the requirement of a macronutrient in a meal and add one in. I recommend using the extensive macronutrient list on the RP app that you can download from your app store on either iOS or Android.

Step 5
Swap for favorable PCF

Now that we have designed a weekly plan for ourselves that includes four to five meals a day and a PCF in each meal, we are miles ahead of the person who downloaded a fitness–influencer's six-week diet to follow.

The next step in the simple stage of nutrition is to swap the macronutrients for what we call "favorable proteins, carbs, and fats." Using something like the RP app, start to swap out macronutrients that are less favorable for some healthier alternatives.

For example, some meats would be considered a protein source; however, they may also be high in fat content such as a Scotch fillet beefsteak. You can simply swap this for a leaner cut or a chicken breast option. Both are protein sources, one with fewer calories per serving. Another example would be changing from white bread to a more grain-dense bread.

KPIs

The final step of the simple stage is to change unfavorable macronutrients in your four-to-five-meal a day nutrition plan to more favorable PCF choices. This teaches us the flexibility of choice and allows us to identify on a menu or when shopping what is what so that we can make sure we can give ourselves the best possible chance at nailing our plan and our education.

Bonus Step
Go to the next level
Now that you have gone through the five simple steps, it may be time to look ahead at the next developmental stage and really start to build a sustainable nutritional lifestyle.

In the following sections, Nick Shaw will go into depth on the information required to meet the sustainable and specific nutritional stages.

Sustainable, Conscious Eating

By Nick Shaw

I run a fitness/nutrition company called Renaissance Periodization (RP for short or more commonly known as @rpstrength on Instagram). Drawing from my years of helping individually coach over 1,000 clients via one-on-one coaching and also helping hundreds of thousands of clients worldwide via our best-selling RP Diet Templates and e-books I would love to share some further nutrition information that my good friend Dave has touched on.

So if the goal is to be an A+ student, then that is certainly worth aiming for although it is a long and tough process.

You're going to first have to master the basics of nutrition (what are calories, protein, carbohydrates, fats, etc.). It is with this foundation that you can then start to understand how/why things work they do and then you can begin to move up the ladder into more advanced techniques. When I've given seminars, I always like to make training analogies. Suppose you're a first timer walking into a gym, you most likely (if you have a competent coach or somebody guiding you) are NOT going to be working on your snatch on day one. What you should be doing is working on the fundamentals like learning how to move properly and learning the basic lifts with proper form. It is then and only then that you begin to move onto advanced lifts like the snatch or clean and jerk.

The same holds true for nutrition. You must first start with learning the basics, and, luckily, we at RP have a plethora of resources to help folks understand the basics and then work their way up the ladder to finding how it all ties together to create sustainability and simplicity if the user prefers more precision. Ultimately, knowing how many calories you are consuming and how to manipulate that amount up or down based on your goals is going to be much more important than learning when to eat specific foods or which supplements to take. Let's take a closer look!

Simple—this is where we start, and if we reference the grading scale, this is recommended for those who would like to be at the C level or below. Now, there's nothing wrong with being a C student in this example. C in this case simply means mastering the basics and aiming for a simpler approach. In my 10+ years in the fitness field this is one of the more common mistakes I've seen. A lot of folks aim for precision when what they ultimately need is an understanding of the basics and focusing on ways to be more consistent. Like with training, if you only follow a diet four to five days out of the week, even the greatest diet won't amount to much without consistency. Let's talk about the simple fundamentals of nutrition, and this is a bit of an excerpt from *Understanding Healthy Eating* written by my colleague Dr. Mike Israetel.

What Are Calories?

In the very simplest sense, calories are just a unit with which to measure energy, specifically the energy people get from eating food. When any food that can be used for energy is absorbed after digestion (proteins, carbs, fats, and some other compounds like alcohols), it can be used as energy, fueling the various processes that not only allow for physical activity but that also keep you alive. If you have already consumed enough energy to meet all your needs, almost all foods that have calories can be converted and stored as body fat. So if you eat significantly more calories than you need to fuel your body and its activity on a regular basis, you'll begin to gain fat and, of course, the body weight that fat adds. On the other hand, if you chronically under eat food, the insufficient level of calories means your body will have to go elsewhere to meet its energy needs. If you are working out hard on a regular basis, especially with weights, most of that energy will come from stored body fat, and you'll get leaner. If you don't work out much and still under eat, the losses will come from both muscle and fat. If taken too far, muscle losses can lead to weakness and some health problems (we will get to that in just a bit). For now, just think of calories as "how much food" you are eating. Consume less than you need to fuel your body and you lose weight, consume more and you will gain weight, mostly in the form of body fat.

Calories and Bodyweight

By representing the raw materials and energy needed to keep all our vital systems functioning, calories are critical to life and, of course, by that extension, health. One of the most replicated and well-supported findings through the history of nutrition research is that calorie balance is the *only*, and we mean *only* determining factor of your long-term body weight. You can eat only very special foods, you can time your nutrient intake to the minute, and you can take all the newest supplements, but the only determinant of your body weight will be the balance between how many calories you take in and how many you expend. If you want to lose weight, whatever else you do, you'll have to either lower your calorie intake or raise your physical activity to expend more calories. If you want to maintain weight, you must make sure that on average, you are eating enough food to meet your needs and not much more or less. If you are gaining weight, it's because you are either eating too much food, not being active enough, or both. But hold on, we thought this was a book about health, not bodyweight. What do the two have to do with each other?

Healthy Protein Basics

Because our bodies cannot construct amino acids (the building blocks of body proteins) from just any kind of other calories, they need to be taken in at minimal doses from the diet for both life and health. Aminos (amino acids) rarely occur free form and almost always appear in our food as the building blocks of proteins. When we eat those foods, the proteins are broken down inside our digestive tracts to give us the amino acids we need for our survival and health needs. But all proteins are not the same.

Proteins differ on two main factors and a third factor of protein sources, which also affects health.

All proteins can be ranked on their completeness of digestion. When you eat any protein source, a certain amount of the protein will get digested, making the amino acids broken down usable by the body. However, every protein source will not digest 100 percent completely, and some protein will escape digestion and be excreted out of the body. This results in the amino acid escaping use by our bodies for its essential functions. If we rank all common food protein sources on how big of a proportion of their content gets fully digested and absorbed from the average meal, we find that nearly all animal proteins have very high digestibility, a percentage often in the high nineties. While some plant proteins like soy are just below animal proteins in their completeness of digestion, the average plant-sourced protein is much less digestible than most animal sources. The commonly recognized plant protein known as gluten has been documented with some very low digestion rates, perhaps as low at 25 percent in some cases. This means that if you eat 100 g of protein from a source heavy in gluten, you might only see 25 g of that in your bloodstream as amino acids, and thus only benefit from 25 g of it.

All proteins can be ranked not only on how completely they digest, but on the ratio of amino acids they provide. To the human body, amino acids are like differently shaped building blocks. We need a wide spectrum of them, but because of the specific designs of our own body proteins (which are built by the aminos we eat), we need more of some than others. How closely eaten proteins match up in amino acid fractions with human needs is a ranking that is independent of (and is done after) protein digestibility. Some proteins provide a mixture of aminos that are very close to human needs, while others provide proteins that have way too many aminos of a kind we already have in abundance (not a health risk, just gets burned up for energy or stored as fat instead of built into structures) and not enough of a kind we need more of. When a protein has all of the amino acids in requisite amounts to meet basic survival and health needs, it's called a "complete" protein. When two proteins must be eaten together to fill in each other's gaps of amino insufficiency, they are called "complementary" proteins because they complement each other. Lastly, when a protein source doesn't have all of the needed amino acids in high enough concentrations to support human life and health, it's termed an "incomplete" protein. While all animal sources are complete, most plant sources are not. While some plant sources can form complementary intake pairs with each other (beans and rice being common examples), most plant proteins are classified as incomplete protein sources.

In addition to carrying a significant amount of completely digestible and complete proteins, animal products are also rich in a number of vitamins and minerals that plants tend to have in much smaller quantities or nearly not at all. Examples include some of the B vitamins (in particular B_{12}) and iron.

The whole picture that emerges for protein intake is one that seems to favor the consumption of animal protein sources to best support health. If you don't consume animal protein sources, can you still be maximally healthy? Absolutely, but you need to make sure to take some extra steps to ensure your health, particularly the following:

Focusing your consumption on complete plant sources like quinoa and soy.

Making sure to take in more protein than is recommended for the general meat-eating public to offset the poorer digestion and amino acid fractions of plant proteins.

Consider supplementation with some of the micronutrients inadequately supplied by plant-based diets, such as the B vitamins and iron.

Healthy Carb Basics

When comparing the sources of carbohydrates by their effects on health, we can order them by how they rank on three distinct variables.

Concentration of the micronutrients: fiber, vitamins, minerals, and phytochemicals. Fiber is a type of carbohydrate that we cannot digest (so it has no calories), but it has numerous health benefits, including the lowering of cholesterol levels and controlling spikes in blood glucose. We need vitamins and minerals in minimum doses to survive, and without enough of them, optimal health cannot be attained. Lastly, phytochemicals are special molecular structures found only in plants. While they are not essential to life, many phytochemicals so far discovered have a very small but positive effect on human health. When we consider that there are hundreds of documented phytochemicals and that more of them are discovered every year, their health benefits can add up to a still small but meaningful positive effect.

Rank on the Glycemic Index: How quickly and to what magnitude a carbohydrate digests and appears in the blood is represented on the glycemic index. All carb sources can be ranked on the index, which stretches from pure glucose on one end (score 100, meaning a rapid appearance of a lot of glucose in the blood after eating) to pure fiber on the others (score 0, meaning no appearance). What does the magnitude of carb digestion imply for health? By itself, not much. Correlation of the glycemic index to health outcomes has shown some favoritism toward low-glycemic (slower digesting) foods, but not the kind of overwhelming and clear relationship we'd be comfortable making recommendations on. However, lower glycemic foods are slightly healthier in most cases than higher glycemic foods for at least three indirect reasons. First, low glycemic foods almost always tend to be the kinds that have the most fiber and vitamins, minerals, and phytochemicals. Fiber slows down digestion and the subsequent release of glucose into the bloodstream, making it directly responsible for lowering the glycemic index score of any accompanying carbohydrates. Most high-fiber foods are the very plant foods loaded with vitamins, minerals, and phytochemicals. Secondly, because of their slow digestion rates, low-glycemic foods are more likely to provide a steady stream of energy to your daily activities rather than the high-then-crash potential of high-glycemic foods. By providing a steady stream of energy, low-glycemic foods help to support both more stable mental abilities for work and more stable energy levels for continual physical activity through the day, which is itself directly health promoting. Lastly, low-glycemic foods are usually (though not always) more satiating (creating a feeling of fullness) than higher glycemic index foods. And satiation is our third variable for carbohydrate source consideration.

All eaten carbs (and any foods, actually) can be ranked on a scale of satiety promotion. That is, we can answer the question of what kind of carb sources tend to keep you fuller longer, and what kind of other carb sources leave you hungry shortly after eating them. Because the kinds of carbs that, calorie for calorie, lead to more fullness also lead to less overall calorie consumption, they tend to have better effects on health, be it indirectly through the priority of calorie balance.

Taken together, the three considerations for carb source actually lead to simpler diet advice than would initially seem when you consider having to juggle the net agreement of three different variables. In nearly every case, the healthiest carb sources (as measured by their fulfilment of the above three considerations) are almost always whole grains, fruits, or vegetables. Whole grains, fruits, and veggies are jam packed with vitamins, minerals, phytochemicals, and fiber; they are usually lower on the glycemic index than other carb sources; and nearly always cause greater satiety due to their high fiber and water concentrations giving them large, stomach-expanding volumes. Because processing strips off some fiber, water, vitamins, minerals, and phytochemicals, the healthiest kinds of carbs tend to be the least processed kind. While carbs like lactose sourced from dairy are by no means bad for health, most individuals would see the biggest health benefits by focusing their carb intakes on whole grains, fruits, and vegetables.

Healthy Fat Basics

There are four basic categories of fat, based on their molecular structures. While we won't dive into the details of those structures, here's a basic synopsis of each kind of fat:

Trans-saturated fats, or *trans fats*, are fats most commonly used to increase the shelf life of common baked goods. Diets high in trans fats have been shown to be deleterious to health, particularly to cardiovascular health. The recommended intake of trans fats is "minimal," and luckily their use in food prep in modern countries has been in fast decline.

Saturated fats are most commonly found in animal products like fatty steak, dairy products, butter and cheese in particular. While they are not bad for health in moderation, their consumption in excess has been associated with slightly poorer health outcomes, particularly for cardiovascular disease.

Polyunsaturated fats are most commonly found in plant oils (like corn oil), but are found in animal sources as well. Consumption of polyunsaturated fats in moderation doesn't harm health, and, in fact, two types of polyunsaturated fats (omega-3 and omega-6) are essential to survival and health because we can't make them ourselves and must get them from our diets. While we need both omega-3 and omega-6 fats in our diets, most of us in the modern west get plenty of omega-6 but sometimes not enough omega-3. It has been shown that grass-fed animals have higher concentration of omega-3 fats in their meats, and it very well might be slightly worth consuming more grass-fed animal products than the alternative. While moderation is the best recommendation for polyunsaturated fats, higher levels of omega-3 fats have been shown to improve cognitive functioning and decrease cardiovascular disease risk.

Monounsaturated fats are a variety of fats that mostly occur in plant foods. Common sources of this fat include nuts, nut butters, olive and canola oils, and avocado. Their positive health effects when they replace saturated or polyunsaturated fats in a diet are incredibly well documented, and if you are going to eat a lot of any one kind of fat, monounsaturated is your best bet.

What this means is that C students are simply after a level of basic understanding that can help them make more and more of the "right" decisions when it comes to food choices. This doesn't mean they need to worry about the finer details, but simply understanding what proteins, carbs, and fats are can help lead to better health/diet outcomes from forming a more basic understanding of which foods are likely better choices than others.

Now that we've covered some basics of nutrition we can start to focus on the more advanced priorities. As we climb up the ladder of priorities, which ironically leads to the priorities that require LESS attention we start to see how they are for the more advanced students seeking grades higher than a C and more like the B range. This is where we tackle things like the importance of the right macronutrient breakdowns and nutrient timing.

When eating for general health, there are typically a lot of ways to eat that arrive at similar outcomes. That means that some folks can eat a higher-carb, lower-fat diet and be entirely healthy. Others can eat a diet that is much lower in carbs and higher in fat and still be healthy. Others may eat more of a carnivore style diet with very high protein (meat) and much lower carbs and fats and still be relatively healthy. The same can be said of folks who enjoy a vegan diet with no meat. How can we have similar health outcomes with diets that are so different? The key here is recognizing the power of calories from the previous excerpt and seeing how powerful that is. So long as calories are controlled for, individuals can enjoy a wide variety of different macronutrient breakdowns and still reach similar health outcomes.

As we search for more details in our quest to conquer nutrition, we turn to an excerpt from *The Renaissance Diet 2.0* e-book written by my colleagues to understand how specific macronutrient distributions can start to enhance body composition results, and as you aim to be a "higher achiever" focusing on more of these smaller details can start to add up.

The following figure is our pyramid that represents the most important factors in successful dieting to reach body composition goals. As mentioned before, calorie balance (how many calories you consume versus how many you burn) is the top priority in this as well as for healthy eating.

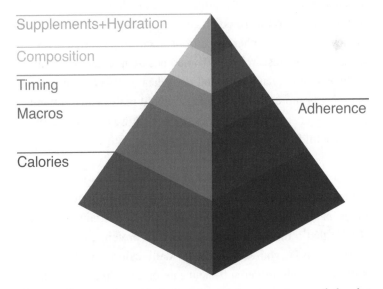

The Diet Priority Pyramid depicts the relative importance of the diet priorities for body composition and performance outcomes. (Credit to Eric Helms and his team for the pyramid organization of nutritional priorities. We highly recommend their Muscle and Strength Pyramid books).

Minimum, Maximum, and Recommended Daily Protein Intake

We have two means of establishing maximum protein intake. The first is to ask whether some amount of dietary protein can be toxic. Proteins need to be broken down into the constituent molecules, and many of the by-products are processed by the kidneys. Though an important consideration, both theoretical supposition (what volumes of protein breakdown would be required to overtax the kidneys) and direct evidence from carefully controlled research, point to the same conclusion: There appears to be no realistic protein amount that is dangerous for human consumption (this of course excludes individuals with kidney disease or other conditions requiring restricted protein intake). Recent research tested outcomes of up to 2 g per pound of body weight per day and found no ill health effects. This amount is probably more than most people would realistically eat on any diet that accounted for macronutrients anyway, so it is not the most useful figure in determining protein maxima.

The second means of establishing a top end for protein intake comes from caloric constraint and the need for minimum intake of other macronutrients. It is from the caloric constraint hypothesis (CCH) that a more applicable maximum protein amount comes. Very simply, if you eat *all* of your daily calories in protein, you will not be able to get sufficient fats or carbohydrates and your health, sport performance, and recovery will suffer. Maximum protein intake is as much protein as can be eaten within the caloric constraint while still allowing the minimum amounts of fat and carbohydrate for health.

Somewhere between this and the minimum protein needed lies an optimal range of intakes. It would be great if we could recommend one minimum protein intake amount that would fit all dietary needs. Unfortunately, the minimum protein to support health differs from the minimum amount of protein needed to gain muscle, and so on. In order to calculate the appropriate range, assessing protein minima for various purposes (health and various specific sports) is required.

Protein Needs for General Health

The minimum amount of daily protein needed for health is about 0.3 g of protein per pound of body weight. Note that this minimum is not a recommendation for physique or performance; it is the minimum needed *just* for health.

Current research cannot agree on a specific value of protein intake for best health. Some studies have suggested that better health comes from a lower-protein diet, but these conclusions were probably not the best interpretation of the data. When variables such as saturated fat intake or overly processed food consumption are accounted for in literature reviews, it appears that individuals who eat mostly whole food diets that include high protein are just as healthy as their low-protein counterparts (and likely have better physiques). It does seem that the consumption of a minimum of 0.3 g of protein per pound of body weight per day can support good health, at least for nonathletes and relatively sedentary individuals.

On the other hand, higher protein intakes support greater muscle masses, which can potentiate higher activity levels, greater resistance to injury, and better long-term health. Eating more protein has also been shown to enhance satiety (the feeling of fullness) for longer than carbs or fats in calorically equivalent amounts. Obesity has negative health effects that can lead to diabetes, cardiovascular disease, and other comorbidities that can be prevented or ameliorated by weight loss. Raising protein intake may therefore make dieting easier and enhance weight loss in obese individuals, indirectly improving health. Increased protein consumption can also increase lean body mass in old age, which is positively correlated with longevity, the ability to exercise later in life, and resistance to injury in older age—all relevant to long-term health.

These indirect benefits are extremely valuable and should be taken into consideration in the big picture of health choices. Even if one can get by acutely on lower protein diets, long-term health is likely benefited by the daily consumption of more than 0.3 g protein per pound of body weight.

At this time the data suggest a range of between 0.3 g and 2.0 g of protein per pound of body weight per day as best for health—though we suspect that the low end of this range may not be ideal for long-term health and independence in old age. Athletes should likely lean toward a range of 0.8 g to 2.0 g of protein per pound of body weight per day to support lean body mass maintenance for sport performance.

Minimum, Maximum, and Recommended Daily Carbohydrate Intake

Glucose can be obtained from other macronutrients, albeit less efficiently. The human body does not actually need any carbohydrates from the diet for basic survival and health. So the minimum carbohydrate intake could be set at zero. The most abundant sources of needed vitamins, minerals, phytochemicals, and fiber, however, are vegetables, fruits, and whole grains, all of which contain carbs. While most of these micronutrients can be supplemented, many are absorbed more efficiently when consumed via whole foods, so eliminating carbs entirely presents some risk to health.

How much plant-based food must be consumed to meet micronutrient needs for health depends on which foods are consumed. If a high diversity of colorful veggies and fruits are eaten regularly, the micronutrients they contain will satisfy health requirements with relatively low carb intakes. On the other hand, if more processed grains are the primary source, a considerably higher amount of carb-rich food must be eaten to ensure adequate micronutrient intake.

The ceiling for carbohydrate intake is best set by using CCH to dictate carb amounts once protein and fat are at their respective minima. Within this constraint, there is no notable downside to very high carb consumption. These recommendations are fairly vague, so we will outline some specifics for carb intake below.

Carbohydrate Needs for Health

In our estimate, if the predominant carb sources in the diet are vegetables and fruit, a minimum of around 0.3 g of carbs per pound of body weight per day is sensible for vitamin and micronutrient intake needs. Though currently popular, ketogenic diets are not ideally healthy.

Many of the conclusions regarding the benefits of ketogenic diets have been determined in studies using obese subjects, for whom any means of weight loss leads to improved health. Better studies are needed in healthy but sedentary individuals for a full assessment of the benefits and downsides to low-carb eating. For short periods of time (months), ketogenic diets might be safe, but they are not recommended for health in the long-term (years). This is different for people who eat a ketogenic diet for medical reasons, a topic that is being widely researched.

Direct study of the subject and decades of research on individuals who eat vegan or otherwise highly plant-based diets have shown that relatively high-carb consumption has no negative health effects on its own. Remember, though, that we are viewing all these statements through the lens of the CCH. If you are eating so many carbs that you begin to violate your calorie needs and gain excessive fat, negative health effects will almost certainly follow. On the other hand, if you displace too much fat and protein with carb calories, you will also likely suffer negative health effects. Within these CCH-based constraints, even the maximum amount of carbohydrate consumption in no way interferes with health. For example, many vegans regularly consume upward of 80 percent of their calories from carbohydrates, and as a group, they tend to be just about as healthy as any group ever studied.

The important exceptions to this rule are of course individuals who have conditions related to blood sugar regulation, such as diabetics, individuals with thyroid issues, or polycystic ovary syndrome (PCOS), and many people with chronic digestive illnesses and other metabolic disorders. For any diet change they wish to make, a consultation with their medical doctor or clinical nutritionist (registered dietician in the United States) is essential.

Because vegetable, fruit, and whole grain consumption is so supportive of optimal health, we do not recommend carbohydrate intakes of much less than 0.5 g per pound of body weight per day for most people in the long term. This minimum can be dropped to 0.3 g per pound of body weight per day if carb sources are all whole food fruits and vegetables—to get enough micronutrients for best health. Remember that these relatively low needs for health are not adequately supportive of sport performance or muscle retention and that carb levels must be increased for best fitness outcomes.

When considering the nutritional content for this book, we decided against offering up nutritional plans due to the fact that people have different needs and different goals and are at different stages of their life. We recommend you take this knowledge and apply it and see how you go. The other offer for those of you who want a more specific personal template is to go to https://renaissanceperiodization.com/diet-templates and download the RP app from the app store and start your two-week free trial.

No matter which path you decide to go down, we recommend that you keep learning and keep applying the rules offered in this book.

Specific Eating Standards

By Nick Shaw

This stage of development is, as the title offers, more specific. People in this stage are likely to be at the peak stage of their development or chosen sport. As mentioned earlier, when people jump from a low grading to attempt this level, they often fall back to their lower level. We have to work through all the levels to get here and also understand whether or not we need to get to this level in the first place.

For a lot of people, this level isn't necessarily unattainable; it's more so that it isn't necessary for their goals. Once again, it is being mindful of where we are, where we want to go, and what do we need to do to get there.

Carbohydrates in Performance and Body Composition Enhancement

The nervous system relies heavily on glucose; so much so that large rapid drops in blood glucose can cause failures in brain function and even death. The nervous system can use other fuel sources, like the ketones that are produced from fat and protein during times of low carbohydrate intake, but this is your body's "emergency only" backup.

Normal blood glucose levels sustain mental acuity, force production, and fatigue prevention. Brain cells are well fed and very responsive when glucose is readily available in the blood. This means that reaction times are quicker, decision making is sharper, and motivation is higher.

When blood glucose is too low, nervous system operation can falter leading to fewer motor units (parts of a muscle all connected to one nerve) contributing to a muscle contraction. This in turn leads to lower contractile force and less strength, speed, power, and endurance.

Falling blood glucose levels have been shown consistently to correlate with rising levels of fatigue. Tough competitions lead to mental and physical fatigue naturally, but low blood sugar hastens this fatigue. Maintaining blood glucose levels through carbohydrate consumption during sport training or competition can therefore delay the onset of fatigue.

Glucose is also the preferred fuel for high-intensity or voluminous physical exertion. Repetitive exertions of over 30 percent of the muscle's maximum contraction force rely primarily on carbohydrates, particularly muscle glycogen. Nearly all sports require high levels of force exertion. While many sports are characterized in part by lower-intensity exertions, it is often the magnitude of the high-intensity components that determines positive performance. This is particularly true for any style of weight training. There is an argument that singles (sets of one repetition) do not require much carbohydrate, and this is true at the acute level. Singles and doubles rely on stored ATP and creatinine phosphate for energy. (For those of you who are more detailed- and scientific-minded, ATP stands for Adenosine Triphosphate. Now you know.) These contractions are still initiated by the nervous system, and thus dietary carbohydrate still benefits them even if high glycogen stores specifically do not. In addition, the recovery of ATP and creatinine phosphate stores after each set relies on carbohydrates. In any case, repeated sets and any repetitions over three get a significant proportion of their energy needs via glycogen so almost all weight-training styles, in addition to almost all sports, rely on carbohydrate for maximum performance.

Consuming carbohydrates is an extremely powerful means of preventing muscle loss. Carbs provide an energy source that prevents the breakdown of tissue for fuel. In addition, anabolism is achieved via both glycogen- and insulin-mediated pathways, both of which are directly affected by carb intake. Elevations in blood glucose resulting from carbohydrate consumption lead to the secretion of insulin, a highly anabolic hormone. Although insulin is anabolic to both muscle *and* fat tissue, for leaner individuals doing resistance training, the net effect of insulin is biased toward building muscle tissue more than fat tissue. Like many other hormones (be it testosterone, growth hormone, estrogen, etc.), insulin exerts most of its power when its concentration is chronically elevated. If insulin is high post workout for an hour but very low during the rest of the day, the total exposure of the muscles to insulin is relatively insignificant. If insulin is instead elevated for a large portion of each day, its anabolic and anticatabolic signaling effects can add up to make substantial differences in muscularity over the long (months) term.

While protein elevates insulin to some extent, fat does not elevate insulin much or at all. Carbohydrate consumption on the other hand has a predictable, consistent effect on blood insulin levels. If elevating insulin for muscle growth is the goal, then eating carbs is the easiest and most effective path.

Glycogen-mediated anabolism is perhaps even more important to muscle gain and retention. Eating carbs allows you to train harder, which grows more muscle and diverts more calories toward muscle repair and upkeep. When this is done on a hypocaloric diet, it has the potential to cancel the catabolism stimulated by insufficient calorie intake. Additionally, it has been repeatedly shown that training under low-glycogen conditions (resulting from low carb eating) leads to more muscle loss than training under high-glycogen conditions. Multiple molecular pathways for these effects have also been elucidated, so both the effect and mechanism have been well studied. In other words, if you chronically undereat carbs, you will almost certainly gain less muscle on hypercaloric diets and lose more during hypocaloric phases.

Minimum, Maximum, and Recommended Daily Fat Intake

Fat Needs for Health

Minimum fat requirements are uniform irrespective of activity level and are matched for health and sport outcomes. The minimum recommendation is around 0.3 g per pound of body weight per day—this amount makes it very likely that enough essential fats (Omega-3 and Omega-6 fats) will be consumed to meet minimum needs. In addition, this minimum value ensures enough fat intake to support sufficient testosterone, estrogen, and prostaglandin production for best body composition and performance outcomes. As with other nutrients, there is some variance in this value based on the individual; 0.3 g per pound of body weight per day covers almost all individuals in most circumstances. In terms of maximum fat intake, current science suggests that as long as fats are not so high as to violate the CCH for carbs, proteins, and calories, the amounts eaten within these constraints can be considered healthy. There is some evidence to suggest that keeping calorie contribution from fat under 40 percent of total daily calories might be better for gut health and body composition, so this is a sensible maximum to consider within caloric constraints. What types of fats and in what ratios they are consumed can alter health and body composition outcomes.

It must be noted that some individuals will have slightly better bloodwork at lower or higher fat intake levels. If health is your number-one priority, trying different ranges and assessing your health with a medical professional via bloodwork is likely a good idea. This means that some people might be able to have a diet that meets minimum carb, protein, and micronutrient needs and is relatively high in fat and still be very healthy. Some prerequisites in quality of food sources would have to be met on such a diet, but it is within the realm of possibility.

Unfortunately, such a diet is not optimal for performance or body composition changes.

Fats in Performance and Body Composition Enhancement

The production of testosterone and estrogen relies, in part, on fat intake and both of these hormones are critical to muscle gain, muscle retention, and nearly all performance adaptations. In addition, fat intake supplies essential fatty acids for the production of physiologically active lipid compounds that play key roles in the regulation of muscle growth and repair, particularly through their mediation of inflammatory processes.

Some have argued for fats as a primary fuel source for athletic performance, most recently ultra-endurance performance. Proponents of this often argue that such performance benefits are not truly realized until an individual becomes "fat adapted" (by staying away from carbohydrates almost entirely for weeks on end). As of this writing, there is very little evidence that fat is a high-performance fuel and a wealth of evidence that carbohydrates are the better performance fuel source. As important as fats are, they are not the best performance fuel, and so recommendations for fat consumption ranges for sport are very similar to those for general health. CCH based on sport and recommendations for compliance on particular diet phases do alter these recommendations slightly, and these are discussed below.

As you can see and as you would expect to become a better "student," there are more details and specific variables that need to be accounted for when it comes to your macronutrient breakdown in regard to not only eating for health, but also for general body composition improvement. Because calories are constrained and cannot be infinite (DANG IT!), we have to work within the constraints and for any increase in one macronutrient another one must go down to offset the difference. The figure goes over the CCH.

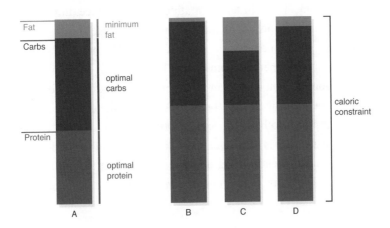

A: Protein, carb, and fat ratios when protein is set at its optimum. B, C, and D: The relative carb and fat deficiencies that can result from overeating protein within a given caloric constraint.

What this means in the big picture is that as we get more advanced, it's beneficial to be careful about how the macronutrient breakdown and distribution impacts your specific goals. The more general your goals are, the more flexible you can be in your approach. As you approach the best "students" out there, the need to focus on the details increases and requires a more rigorous examination of how everything interacts in terms of what you eat and even when you eat it!

So you want to be a 4.0 student, right? You had better master the previous pages in understanding eating for not only general health, but also for body composition and performance goals. At the top of aforementioned pyramid are a couple other smaller/minor priorities. Things like nutrient timing, food composition, and supplement intake.

Not only are the details important for those students looking to be a 4.0 student, but in terms of athletic performance, things like nutrient timing and supplement intake can make a substantial impact as you compete at the highest levels. The need for details when you're competing against other talented individuals who are just as good as you can mean a few percentage points difference. It may not seem like much, but consider what the difference is at the Olympics or other high-level sporting events. The difference in a 100 m race is tenths or even hundredths of seconds. The difference at a weightlifting or powerlifting meet may only be a couple of kilograms. Those details can add up!

For each of these minor priorities, we will give a quick chapter summary from the *RP Diet 2.0* e-book instead of diving too deep into the details here:

Nutrient timing describes how calories and macronutrients are assigned relative to time throughout the day. Factors of nutrient timing include meal number, meal spacing, meal size, meal macro content, meal food composition, and timing around physical activity.

Nutrient timing manipulations may not be nearly as powerful as calorie or macronutrient manipulations, but they still provide a tangible and practical benefit to enhancing body composition and performance.

Daily protein intake should be divided into four to eight meals across the day, each containing one-eighth to a quarter of total daily protein.

The larger the meals and more slowly digested, the longer the following intermeal interval will be, but extremely large or small meals should be avoided.

Daily carbohydrate intake should be biased toward activity periods, with the largest doses generally occurring in the pre-, intra-, and post-training time periods.

Daily fat intake should be biased away from activity periods and biased toward longer periods without regular meals such as sleep or while at work.

Slow-digesting protein should be the core of your bedtime meal.

Extreme timing manipulations that sacrifice your daily calories, macros, or sleep quality are not recommended. The latter variables are more impactful to your physique and performance.

Food composition describes the quality of food in terms of its digestibility, digestion rate, and the content of micronutrients and fiber.

The quality of protein is largely determined by the essential amino acid profile and its digestibility and to a smaller extent by its micronutrients content.

The quality of carbohydrate is primarily determined by the digestion rate, or how quickly it can be absorbed into the bloodstream, and its micronutrient and fiber content.

The quality of fat is primarily determined by the class of fat, and diets should generally prioritize monounsaturated fats, polyunsaturated fats, and saturated fats, in that order, while keeping trans fat consumption to a minimum.

A well-balanced diet will generally meet all of the daily micronutrient requirements; however, during hypocaloric periods and periods where certain macronutrients are deprioritized, a vitamin supplement can help ensure micronutrient values are met.

The previous chapter summary is not to dismiss the importance of eating a well-rounded diet, but it should be noted that this is in relation to eating for losing fat, gaining muscle, and improving sport performance. The last bullet point sums it up best. Generally speaking, a well-rounded diet focusing on primarily whole foods like lean proteins, fruits and vegetables, healthy carb sources, and healthy fat sources is a great start for anybody from a C student all the way up to an A+ student.

Last, but certainly not least, in terms of popularity for nutrition are supplements and hydration!

Drinking to slake thirst is sufficient to meet most people's hydration needs, though circumstances involving high sweat output or exercising in the heat may require more deliberate hydration routines.

Urine color and body weight changes are simple tools that can be used to assess degrees of dehydration.

Excessive water intake, particularly without electrolytes, can lead to hyponatremia.

The vast majority of dietary supplements have no supported effects, and even the most effective contribute minimally to fitness outcomes.

The supplements with the most support for body composition, performance, and health are caffeine, whey protein, casein protein, creatinine, carbohydrate formulas, multivitamins, and omega-3s.

Your homework is complete! You now have a solid summary on some of the intricacies as it relates to dieting for general health as well as improving body composition and performance. Just remember, the more general the goals you have the more relaxed and flexible you can be in your approach. Just as you would imagine getting an A+ requires a lot of hard work via studying and homework, the same applies for those who want to master all the nutritional priorities ranging from health to performance goals.

I would like to thank my colleagues for all their hard work in the two books that were referenced in this section. If you would like to read more about eating for general health, check out our book *Understanding Healthy Eating*. If you want to read much, much more about eating for fat loss, muscle gain, and/or improving performance, please check out *The Renaissance Diet 2.0*. Thanks again to my good friend Dave Nixon for letting me contribute to his book!

* * *

When considering the nutritional content for this book, we decided against offering up nutritional plans due to the fact that people have different needs and different goals and are at different stages of their lives. We recommend you take this knowledge and apply it and see how you go. The other offer for those of you who want a more specific personal template, go to https://renaissanceperiodization.com/diet-templates or download the RP app from the app store and start your two-week free trial.

No matter which path you decide to go down, we recommend you keep learning and keep applying the rules offered in this book.

While writing this book, it dawned on me that the information that both Nick and I could relay in both the nutrition and the training subjects was at a point where it could be its own book. Throughout, I wanted to continually give insight into how we can best address all three areas of health with our mind and use practical and objective information to apply to our day to day life in the form of training programs or nutritional plans. With this new awareness, I wanted to ensure that I could provide as much developmental work as possible in this edition. As for actual nutrition and training plans, we decided against just giving out any old plan considering the vast range of people who will pick this book up and read it, and they will all have different goals, different restrictions, and different life conditions. There is a free GPP training download at bossfit.online that you can start with as well as a vast range of other programs that are more tailored for your goals and the type of training that most interests you. As for your nutrition plan, as stated previously, you should use the two-week free trial for the RP app that can get you started and well on your way to developing your own specific nutrition plan.

One of the most important things when it comes to nutrition is the education and the execution of a meal plan. Vague plans give vague results. In saying that, we have to start somewhere. Nick and I wanted to offer some of the best information from both a nutritional research and a psychological viewpoint. If you are wanting to take your nutritional education to the next stage, then I highly recommend investing in it. Of course, I recommend RP, but I am fully aware that there are multiple credible and professional educators and coaches in the industry. Once again, do your homework and due diligence and find a course or a coach that best fits you and where you are at.

PART IV

The
THREE-YEAR
LETTER

One of my favorite spots in America is Hermosa Beach. I remember telling some of my American friends this, and they laughed. Of course, I know there are some amazing spots all across America, but for some reason, Hermosa had my vibe and was what I needed at the time I first went there.

My first trip to America was when I was 26. I decided to tour the United States and go to a heap of different gyms, blogging my experience. My first training tour consisted of Gym Jones in Salt Lake City, Bobby Maximus, Chris Duffin, C. T. Fletcher, The CrossFit Games, Westside Barbell, and my good friend Jay Maryniak.

I left Sydney airport with 2,000 thousand Australian dollars in my pocket for a month in America with only three nights of accommodation booked. So, by the time I had booked a hostel in Hermosa after a couple of rough weeks, I was short on cash and short on morale. I had no idea how I was getting out of there and was hoping some money would come through in the next couple of days from a tax return.

One morning while I was at the hostel in Hermosa Beach, I opened up my e-mail inbox to an e-mail I received from a client back home. In short the e-mail was informing me of her recent successful ski trip to Japan. Although I had been thanked before for helping people achieve their goals this one really stood out for me. On reflection it may have had something to do with being low on morale and receiving an endorphin boost, but what I really think it had more to do with was the fact that this person was able to build memories with her family. Her discipline to her training wasn't to get rid of knee pain; it was to create more memories with her family. For her to do that, she had to participate more, in order for her to participate more, she had to reduce her knee pain.

This was really the birth of the three-year letter for me. This client was training in the vicinity of about 18 months at the time, and she is still training with us to the day of writing this four years later. What dawned on me during this time was just how important and intergenerational her achievement was. We all remember what our caretakers did or didn't do with us, and it impacted us. It was more than just skiing, it was living.

This is when I saw more value in long-term progression over short-term results. Everything worth achieving is worth working for.

What will your three-year letter say from today?

If I could offer you one more exercise before I sign off it would be this: write a letter to yourself today as if it were you in three years' time. Include what you are grateful for, include what you have achieved, include your future aspirations, and send it to yourself via e-mail. If you want to get super fancy, then set a reminder for three years' time to go back to that e-mail and read over it. Another option would be to handwrite it and put it in a safe storage box somewhere in the house. At some stage in the future, you will come past it again be it when you move or are cleaning up. Either way, invest in three-year letters, not eight-week challenges.

To reiterate the core message from this book, always continue to invest in your HIQ and, most importantly, your Self.

Tambra to me: **July 17, 2015, 9:23 PM**

Hi Dave,

Skiing went well, I broke my record of six consecutive days skiing—I achieved eight! What's more I did not pull up too sore. I think there are a number of things that have helped; because of my strength my technique has improved, which means so has my skiing ability. Had conditions been better this trip, I would have given some of the intermediate runs a crack, but, hey, the season is only beginning :) Next time we come, more of the runs and lifts will be open, and I will be able to achieve my goal of skiing in and out of the lodge. I did mobility work most days, when I got back with enough time before dinner . . . some days, if I was having a good day on the snow I kept telling myself just one more run . . . which meant I would get back a bit late.

Anyway, I am really happy with the way everything is going—skiing is so much better when you feel like you are in control and can feel the snow. Thank you!

I hope all is going well with your holiday, I am enjoying reading your daily updates.

Tambra

Credits

Cover & interior design: Annika Naas
Layout: Amnet Services

Illustrations: © Dave Nixon
Part III illustrations: © Renaissance Periodization

Managing editor: Elizabeth Evans
Copyeditor: Amnet Services